Parenting with a Partner with Asperger
Syndrome (ASD)

Out of Mind -
Out of Sight

Practical Steps to Saving You
and Your Family

By
Kathy J. Marshack, Ph.D.

Parenting with a Partner with Asperger Syndrome (ASD)

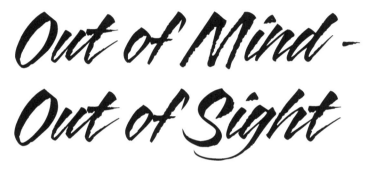

Practical Steps to Saving You and Your Family

By
Kathy J. Marshack, Ph.D.

© 2013 Kathy J. Marshack, Ph.D., P.S.
P.O. Box 873429
Vancouver, Washington 98687
kmarshack@kmarshack.com
www.kmarshack.com / 360-256-0448

Edited By: Janet Herring-Sherman

Cover Illustration: Design by Lisa Archilla

Model Photo, Trees, Family Silhouette: Colourbox.com

Font: Blaze ITC & Minion

ISBN: 1481930885
ISBN 13: 9781481930888

Library of Congress Control Number: 2013900479
CreateSpace Independent Publishing Platform
North Charleston, South Carolina

Publisher's Cataloging-in-Publication

Marshack, Kathy, 1949-

Life with a partner or spouse with Asperger Syndrome: out of mind out of sight: practical steps to saving you and your family / by Kathy J. Marshack.--1st ed.--North Charleston, S.C.: CreateSpace Independent Publishing Platform.

   1. Asperger's syndrome--Patients--Family relationships. 2. People with mental disabilities--Marriage--Parenting. 3. Interpersonal communication. I. Title. II. Title. Out of mind - out of sight.

Table of Contents

Dedication

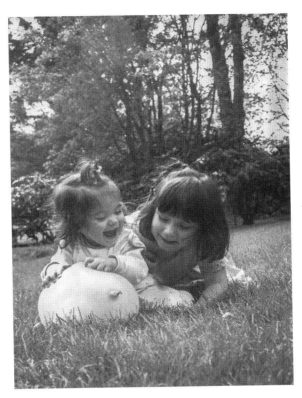

  This book is dedicated to my incredible daughters, Phoebe and
Bianca. Through parenting you, loving you, watching you grow, letting
you go . . . . I learned that I am not alone.

Foreword

It was during my doctoral education at Fordham University that my mentor, Dr. Ernst Vanbergeijk, first introduced me to the unique challenges and needs of parents caring for a child diagnosed with Asperger Syndrome (AS). The trajectory of the lives of a family touched by AS is never predictable. Dr. Kathy Marshack, in her new book, *Out of Mind-Out of Sight*, demonstrates how these lives can, however, be made more manageable and even enjoyable.

Through my research and practice, I have discovered the feelings of exclusion the AS diagnosis can bring to a family. Few outsiders understand the kind of continuous PTSD that AS family members live with. While much information is available today on AS as a diagnosis, it remains a difficult subject to write about. I believe that's because of the irregularities surrounding the AS diagnosis and its treatment: Dr. Marshack succeeds in writing it masterfully.

She uses empathy and fact to bring great integrity to those with Asperger Syndrome and dignity to those impacted by AS. As she did in her first book, *Going Over the Edge? Life With a Partner or Spouse with Asperger Syndrome,* Dr. Marshack uses genuine vignettes (from her private practice) to help the reader walk in the shoes of both the AS and the neurotypical (NT) person living with the AS individual(s).

For me, the beauty of this book is in its sincere concern for everyone on the spectrum and beyond. Although I am an NT interfacing with individuals on the autism spectrum, I have developed my own theory: I suggest that we are all on the autism spectrum to one degree or another.

Dr. Marshack also explores the delicate balance required between an AS and an NT parent, spouse and professional counselor. For those of us who are scientists and researchers constantly seeking evidence to support the existence of concepts or constructs, Dr. Marshack demonstrates the existence of intuition and its importance in our lives. She reminds NTs not to ignore this gut feeling since it can assist us in understanding and, perhaps more importantly, responding compassionately to our loved ones on the spectrum. She encourages NTs to commence a catharsis of feelings in a safe and systematic way.

Many of us do not fully grasp that our environment, too, can influence development. Therefore, the quality of marriage can influence a child's well-being. This is exactly why a vulnerable child can be greatly impacted by their parents' marital dynamic and interactions—and why an AS/NT couple needs to find ways to communicate as best they can. Intuition can go a long way toward helping NTs comprehend the AS environment in which they live and love. Dr. Marshack shows us how by recounting professional and personal encounters.

Dr. Marshack makes a huge contribution in her new book: She urges the NTs among us to meet our Aspies in the context of their lives instead of trying to change them. Many of us do not always, *Stop, Think and Reflect* on what it may feel like to be on the "other side." Yet the way we interpret the context of a situation impacts the way we respond to events in our environment, our lives.

Perhaps, for me, the most profound part of this book is its theoretical foundation. Dr. Marshack introduces modern theory to marshal change in individuals' lives. She accomplishes this by applying clinical terms to real-life scenarios. She makes the book easy-to-use as a reference by concluding each chapter with helpful "Lessons learned" tips and reminders.

Dr. Marshack touches upon the core of what can assist, build and protect the relationships between NTs and Aspies. This book covers everything in an Aspie's life and environment, including cognition, emotion and behavior. It is unique in that it is one of the only books to be so inclusive in its approach to building bridges between Aspies and family members.

Shaping this book, as it did her previous one, is the sacredness of the family unit and its dynamics. With great insight, Dr. Marshack describes the exceptional family dance that Aspies and NTs do. She explains this remarkable dance by emphasizing the main components that define us as human beings: empathy, love and the need for human contact and relationships. Dr. Marshack also explores how the concept of love is not easily or readily understood, explained or expressed by most Aspies. And, she suggests ways for NTs to more accurately interpret their Aspie's actions, or inactions, for the sake of love and well-being.

I hope this book will inspire parents and their children to become more understanding of each other as they go through life's trajectories, or what Dr. Marshack calls a roller coaster ride. At the same time, I hope this innovative, scholarly addition to the body of Aspie literature will begin a new reflection on the mechanics of families with Aspie members.

Dr. Marshack's care and devotion to the Aspie community as a whole is evident in every part of this book. This, coupled with her down-to earth approach to theory, is the reason why this book—perhaps more than any other I have read recently—will have a positive impact in the field of Autism Spectrum Disorders. I am sure this is not the last we will hear from Dr. Marshack, for I'm certain she has many AS/NT stories yet untold.

Oren Shtayermman, Ph.D., M.S.W.
Department of Interdisciplinary Health Sciences
NYIT School of Health Professions
Old Westbury, New York

Preface

I hope this book gets into the hands of parents who really need to know that they are not alone. Parenting with a partner with Asperger Syndrome (AS) or Autism Spectrum Disorder (ASD) is one tough assignment. Many times you feel desperately alone, because your AS spouse, the one person you should be able to confide in, can't read your mind or fathom your feelings. Even worse is the disappointment that comes when you reach out to friends and professionals, who do not comprehend the ongoing traumatic relationship disorder that is the center of your life.

This time, know that you are understood: Every page carries that promise. I have lived this life, too. You may not always be understood in "real time," but through the following pages you can connect with a mom, a daughter, a wife and a psychologist who has lived the life of a neuro-typical (NT) in an Aspie family. This promise provides a pretty good place to start reviving your marriage and your parenting—and claiming personal freedom.

For me, incredible psychological healing came from confronting my fears and writing them down for you. But there was one thing that caused me the greatest struggle in finding my own personal freedom: I had this mental block about the book's cover.

For the life of me, the cover illustration was out of sight and out of mind. When my editor, Janet Herring-Sherman, sent me the final edits, and there was nothing left to write, it dawned on me that this book is about letting go of my role as a parent of two young daughters, one NT and one with Asperger Syndrome.

The girls have grown into young women and are launched into their own lives now. In fact, Phoebe (my NT) has blessed me with my first grandchild. Of course I am still their parent. But I'm no longer the parent of two little girls. I'm no longer the parent struggling with how to reach a child with Asperger Syndrome; and I'm no longer the parent trying to protect an NT child from confusing Aspie behavior and abuse. It is time for me to let go of that chapter of my life and start anew.

Once I'd cleared the mental block about no longer being the mother of two young children, I was open to seeing the book's cover. . . at least the cover that is in my heart if not on the front of this book. I chose an old snapshot of my two children taken in 1991. They were happy and carefree then—before the Asperger's had settled into our lives and taken my breath away. In 1991 my daughters were delightful and inno-cent. I adored them. In this treasured photograph, Phoebe, 15 months old, is on the left. On the right is Bianca, age 4 ½. The moment cap-tured depicts love, the love that goes on forever in my heart—regardless of the heartache that has since transpired. It's a photograph that repre-sents what all parents hope for, well-adjusted children.

Oddly the photograph chose me. Just a few weeks before complet-ing this book, the photo, frame and all, tumbled from its shelf and hit me in the head. I survived, and so did the picture. I placed it back on the shelf, rubbed the bump on my head and thought little of it. I shared the incident with Phoebe, who laughed and suggested there was a story behind it. Indeed there is, and you are holding it in your hands.

As the design of *Out of Mind - Out of Sight* progressed, it became clear that the photo of my two daughters was a perfect fit for the place of honor on the Dedication page. Without my daughters I would never have learned about parenting in a family with an ASD family member.

I would never have learned that I'd grown up with an Asperger mother. I would never have learned how resilient I can be, nor how strong my heart. I would never have reached out to all of you, my international family of NTs parenting with a partner with Asperger Syndrome.

As I close this part of my parenting/life journey, I hope those of you on the path of parenting with a partner with Asperger Syndrome will not feel as alone as I felt. A lot has changed in the more than 20 years since the photo of Phoebe and Bianca as youngsters was taken. Much has been learned about AS. And, yes, there is much more to be discovered. You are part of this second wave of discovery. Your stories are not as unusual as you might imagine. And they're not unheard. I am listening, and I will help you.

Kathy J. Marshack, Ph.D.
Vancouver, WA

Acknowledgments

In this small place at the front of the book, I want to give a huge, heartfelt thank you to all of the wonderful people without whom I could never have finished this book. Many authors struggle to find just the right and most fitting words to convey this debt of gratitude; yet words are not enough. Authors develop intense connections with their supporters. It's inevitable when you walk alongside an author as she pours her soul into a manuscript. Recognition from every corner means a tremendous amount. People who made a passing comment about the book or my work will never know how important that moment in time was to me.

First of course are the many individuals, couples and families who come to life in the book. Through your willingness to tell me your stories I have learned so much. Because of your bravery, others will never have to feel alone: It is the aloneness that is so oppressive. Now readers can take heart, knowing others have gone before you. I have protected the identities of my sources by changing some facts and identifying information. Their stories are a testament to their resilience. It is this resilience that explains everything.

For very personal reasons, my ASD daughter, Bianca, more than anyone, is the main inspiration for this book. Her struggle to discover her talents and her worth taught me so much about staying out of the way instead of hovering. Bianca confounded me time and again. I can't turn back the clock and parent the way I should have. Still, my life with Bianca has taught me to be a better psychologist, a better friend and a better mother. Thank you my beautiful girl.

My younger daughter, Phoebe, has grown into an amazing young woman, who has blessed me with my first grandchild. My heart aches for the heartbreak Phoebe endured living in a family with undiagnosed and untreated Asperger Syndrome. However, she has grown and healed, and I am ever so proud of her resilience. It is gratifying that my NT daughter can take the lessons of our extended family and create a healthier start for her new baby boy.

Three years ago, I started an international Internet support group through www.meetup.com, entitled "Asperger Syndrome: Partners and Family of Adults with ASD," in order to provide a place for parents and partners worldwide to come together and support each other. Currently we have more than 500 members in countries as diverse as Australia, Canada, Dubai, Israel, the United Kingdom, Finland, Germany, New Zealand, South Africa, Nigeria, Brazil, Mexico and America. I am truly touched by the kindness and grace of our members. Each day they reach out to others to offer understanding and support. They share their stories and they listen—they really listen—to the struggles of other NTs. I am amazed at the courage of our members to be there for others when their own struggles are heartbreaking. Please know that this book is written to honor the sacrifices each of you make every day.

I want to extend a thank you to the publisher of my first book on this subject, Keith Myles, and his editor Kirsten McBride. Without your belief in me and my first book, I wouldn't have written a second. Following in your footsteps, my editor for Out of Mind - Out of Sight, Janet Herring-Sherman, helped me produce a manuscript that really speaks to those I want to reach.

I want to thank my wonderful office manager, Michelle Lathim. Michelle has an unwavering devotion to me that can only be explained in one way: She must be an angel. I can still see her earnest expression when she'd said, "Well, the reason that people have such a hard time believing your stories is that they are so unbelievable!" When she'd made that comment, she'd given me a broad smile, as only she can do. We'd both laughed. Yes, Michelle, the stories in this book are unbelievable—but ever so true. It is time they were told.

INTRODUCTION

You Are Not Alone

The roller coaster ride

Parenting with a partner or spouse who has Asperger Syndrome is easier said than done. So, too, has been writing on the subject. The chapters for *Out of Mind - Out of Sight* came together like a roller coaster ride, full of twists and dives. It was much like the experience of a neurotypical (NT)[1] co-parenting with an Aspie. (Aspie is an affectionate term used to describe those who have Asperger Syndrome or AS.) In this book, there are poignant stories of deep despair along with thrilling vignettes of discovery. Just like a roller coaster ride, the topics slam you to attention. You'll recognize: that sinking feeling as you

---

[1]   Neurotypical, or NT, is a popular term used to describe those who are not on the autism spectrum. NTs have good empathy skills and are sensitive to the contexts that surround their relationships. Those with Asperger Syndrome, or Aspies, are defined by their lack of empathy and context blindness. This distinction will become clear as you progress through the book.

plunge into a rapid descent; the sudden jerk that comes with swinging abruptly around a corner; and the thrill/fear of anticipation as you make a slow, grinding ascent, followed by another sheer drop.

I just couldn't find any other way to write this book. I don't believe we need one more quirky, upbeat human interest story on Asperger Syndrome, similar to those in the press these days. Instead, I focus on the harsh realities that an NT faces when co-parenting with an Aspie. I discuss the anguish, fears and losses of the NT parent. I also give you hope and ideas on how to co-parent more successfully. It's important to recognize that revealing the dark side of these relationships enables us to search for solutions to the all-too-real problems of the AS/NT family. The last thing I want to do is leave NT parents feeling that they are alone. Erasing that *aloneness* is the first step toward parenting successfully with an Aspie co-parent.

Out of Mind - Out of Sight has been difficult to write for a very personal reason. I am an NT parent of an Asperger Syndrome child. Writing has been a healing process for me. I worked the outline over again and again, never quite satisfied. I wrote and re-wrote chapters. I scrapped concepts and resurrected them. I took breaks and worked on other things only to be drawn back to finishing this book. Why? As I wrote, I discovered new things about myself and my family, just like peeling away the layers of the proverbial onion. Still, there are many things for me to learn. I certainly hope so, or why be on this remarkable journey on Planet Earth?

One of the differences you will notice between *Out of Mind - Out of Sight* and my previous book, *Going Over the Edge?* is much more of me in these pages. Chapter One, "Helicopter Mother," describes part of my journey with Bianca, my AS daughter. I thought I could remain Dr. Marshack in this book. Try as I might, my professional objectivity kept being infused with my personal experiences. I hope you don't mind. I used my clinical skills, and I researched theories to support my conclusions. Frankly, most of this book was guided by the intuition of a mom who has been there and is there still. I want you to know that you are not alone.

Asperger Syndrome or Autism Spectrum Disorder

Since I first published on the subject of Asperger Syndrome in 2009, there have been many exciting discoveries. This is especially true in the areas of genetics and neuroscience and how they interact with psychology and social learning. I use these discoveries to help make sense of the thoughts, feelings and behaviors of the parents, and children, described in this book. Knowledge is power. The more you know about Asperger Syndrome, the better able you are to parent, co-parent, co-exist and even thrive within your AS/NT family.

As a direct result of integrating science with clinical practice, a professional movement developed to change the name of Asperger Syndrome, or to drop the category entirely. In the 2013 edition of the *Diagnostic and Statistical Manual of Mental Disorders* (DSM-V), leading researchers in the field of autism studies define a new and all encompassing diagnosis, Autism Spectrum Disorder, or *ASD*. The intellectual reasoning for this shift: No two autistic people are the same because of the myriad of unique genetic, personality and environmental factors that come together in one person. With ASD we now have one diagnostic label that encompasses the whole range of what is considered autistic. The concept of a spectrum implies that the diagnosis is varied and multi-dimensional.

What will not change is the basic nature of Autism Spectrum Disorders. ASD is defined as a triad of impairment. Those on the spectrum have difficulties with: (1) social interaction; (2) social communication; and (3) social imitation. However, the depth and breadth of these disabilities is immensely different across the ASD population.

Each Aspie defined under the new diagnosis is as unique as each human being.

The label is changing to incorporate a holistic view of the human condition. In order to bring social science professionals up to speed, the National Institutes of Health (NIH) of the U.S. Department of Health and Human Services launched, in January 2012, an online genetics course for social and behavioral scientists. It's designed to provide education in genetics, so that the scientists can engage in interdisciplinary research with genetics researchers. According to the NIH website, http://www.nih.gov/news/health/jan2012/od-03.htm:

> Increasingly, scientific outcomes are not fully explained by genetic, environmental, or social factors alone or as independent contributors. Instead, public health advances and scientific breakthroughs tend to rely on transdisciplinary teams of social scientists and genetic researchers. This creates a greater need among social and behavioral scientists for an understanding of the complexity of the genetic contribution to health, disease and behaviors.

In *Out of Mind - Out of Sight,* I use the term Asperger Syndrome, or AS, or the colloquial word, "Aspie," because we are familiar with this jargon. Occasionally I will refer to the "spectrum" or "Autism Spectrum Disorder" or even "ASD" to move us along in that direction. I do very much appreciate the more holistic and systemic approach to bringing understanding and healing to the world of AS/NT relationships.

Austen's disconnect

The following anecdote brings out this holistic interplay as I, the psychologist, use knowledge gained from research to guide a young man with ASD toward connecting with his mother.

I first met Austen in the summer before his senior year in high school when he was 17. His parents were frantic: They felt he had only one more school year to become prepared for adult or college life. Austen had been to see lots of psychotherapists over the years. He currently had a very supportive psychiatrist, who managed his medications. Most of Austen's past psychotherapy had consisted of a safe place to talk and feel supported; yet nothing had changed in his behavior. He'd become more and more withdrawn, angry and self-destructive as he approached age 18.

Things were different this visit. I had previously introduced Austen to Neuro-Emotional Technique (NET), a mind-body therapy developed by chiropractor Scott Walker (see: http://www.netmindbody. com/for-patients/an-explanation-of-net). Like hypnosis and some other more holistic therapeutic approaches, NET allows people to bypass conscious, or talk, analysis and get to the heart of their problems. NET enables change without a good explanation for the change. Talk therapy is powerful, of course, but people with Asperger Syndrome often struggle to explain what is going on in their hearts and minds. It is much less stressful for Aspies to use an approach that links talk therapy to change at an unconscious level. Austen is one of those Aspies who benefits from this approach.

Austen arrived one day, ready and eager to share a problem he wanted help with. He said, "I have a problem with my mother. She wants me to clean my bathroom. She even took my laptop away until I clean it."

"Well," I said with a wry smile, "How important is your laptop to you?" I was nudging him to get practical and mind his mom.

"Of course it is vital" Austen quipped, because he knows that I know his world is the Internet. "But that's not the problem I want help with. It's bigger than that."

"Well help me understand the bigger issue Austen. It sort of sounds like a typical power struggle between a teenager and his parent. I mean, I presume your bathroom is a pit," I offered jokingly.

"Oh yes. That is true," Austen agreed. "My bathroom does need to be cleaned for sure! The problem is that I don't do it. It's the 'not doing it' part that stumps me." Austen was describing a complex behavior that could only be defined by Asperger Syndrome. The issue of cleaning his bathroom was indeed more than a childish power struggle.

The light bulb turned on in my mind. "So let me try to understand this Austen. Your bathroom needs cleaning, right? And you would like to get your laptop back, right? But there is this in-between step that is missing for you—the 'not doing it' part. Am I getting your drift?"

"Yes that's it," said Austen, and he perked up. "Of course I want my laptop back, but Mother's taking it away won't make me clean my bathroom. Her actions make no sense to me. I know my bathroom needs cleaning. In fact I want it clean. What's that have to do with my laptop?" Very Aspie logic.

"And do you know how to clean your bathroom? I mean some teenage boys don't know how," I offered while I searched for the missing element.

"No really that's not it. I know how to clean my bathroom, but I don't. It's the 'not doing it' part I need help with." Austen was trying to explain the missing element when he didn't have a word for it.

A second light bulb lit up for me, even brighter than the first. "Austen, I think I got it this time. Let me try to see if this fits. Here are some words for what you are describing. First, you are *motivated* to clean your bathroom because it does need it. You can even understand your mother's demand that you clean it, because it is a pit! And it is your *responsibility*, right?" Austen nods approval. "And you feel a sense of *urgency* to get your laptop back, too. Right?" Austen nods in the affirmative again. "In fact, you would do almost anything to get your laptop back. Right?" One more time Austen is tracking my logic. "It's just that you can't connect cleaning your bathroom and getting the laptop back, because they aren't related. Right?"

"Sure," Austen says. "It is so obvious that these things aren't related, and Mother is always trying this stuff. It never works, so why does she bother?"

I smile with Austen's realization. "Actually, this type of approach is used by lots of parents, and it seldom works with teenagers. We parents think that if we withhold a privilege or a favorite item, we'll get our kids to mind and do things like clean a bathroom. It doesn't work, and all that happens is a power struggle. But let's give Mom some slack here and work out your dilemma."

Austen is ready. I explain, "I think the problem is that we need to connect up your *motivation* to clean your bathroom to your *responsibility* to clean your bathroom with a *call to action* to actually clean your bathroom. That will satisfy the *urgency* you feel to get back your laptop. You'll get a clean bathroom. You can please your mother. She will be motivated to give you back your laptop even though the laptop has nothing to do with a clean bathroom. This is a win-win solution Austen. You already have *motivation*, a sense of *responsibility*, and a feeling of *urgency*. The only thing that is missing for you is a *call to action*. That's the missing piece you keep calling the "not doing it" part. Are you ready to connect the dots?"

Austen's eyes widen, and he smiles. "Yes that's it!" he says. "I am missing the *call to action* part." He raises his arm to begin the process of NET. NET incorporates the concept of Applied Kinesiology, and the meridian system of Chinese medicine. Using acupressure points on the wrist and testing for congruence between mind and body, the patient releases emotional blocks. It's complicated but suffice it to say that

Austen is ready to communicate with his unconscious through NET. Once Austen and I had identified the missing piece, we could use the NET approach to integrate the elements he needed to clean the bathroom. Austen got his laptop back the next day.

Out of mind - out of sight

If you go back and re-read the dialogue between Austen and myself, you may notice that Austen is not motivated by his mother's displeasure with his dirty bathroom. Nor is he motivated by the withholding of his laptop. These are emotional appeals that would require Austen to have an empathically reciprocal relationship with his mother.

In other words, Mom hoped that Austen would want to clean his bathroom because he cares about her opinion of him. When she withheld the laptop, she'd hoped he would connect that she cared about the bathroom's cleanliness as much as he cared about his laptop. These appeals failed, because Austen does not use empathy to make decisions. While he loves his mother, her opinion of him is irrelevant to cleaning the bathroom. He may care about getting his laptop back, but to do so because his mother has feelings about the bathroom literally makes no sense to Austen.

Austen was troubled about why he was not cleaning the bathroom. He was aware a piece of his logic was missing. It's hard for Aspies to discuss what's missing when that piece has never existed for them. I contend that the missing piece in Aspie problem solving is empathy. Out of mind - out of sight. In other words, if the empathy process is not wired into Austen's brain, he can't "see" what to do next. Without empathy, Austen was stymied about how to accomplish something he was powerfully motivated to do.

Empathy is part intuition and part taking action. It is the ability that NTs take for granted when they "just know" what is going on with another person. NTs can take action to "just say" or "just do" the right thing to move a relationship toward mutual understanding and mutual success. Empathy is not really a skill. It is not an object either. Empathy is the

In other words, if the empathy process is not wired into Austen's brain, he can't "see" what to do next. Without empathy, Austen was stymied about how to accomplish something he was powerfully motivated to do.

art of connecting to another person, then back to yourself. By connecting to others, we come to know ourselves, our motives and how we all relate—father to mother, parent to child, brother to sister, friend to friend, neighbor to neighbor, employer to employee. Empathy is so much more than the sum of its parts.

NT children start to develop the art of empathy by age 6: It's not so with Aspies. NT children are wired for this connecting ability called empathy. It naturally unfolds during normal child development. Aspie children, on the other hand, are wired differently: They have to be explicitly and painstakingly taught the traits or parts of empathy—just as I taught Austen about the missing *"call to action"* piece. Learning how to be empathetic does not equate to the reciprocal connecting and relating to others that comes naturally for neurotypicals.

Theorists Simon Baron-Cohen, Adam Smith, Klaus Riegel and Peter Vermeulen are showing us the way toward understanding the differences in the way Aspies and NTs think. Baron-Cohen describes the interpersonal problem for Aspies as zero degrees of empathy. Vermeulen explains further that without empathy Aspies have *context blindness*, or the inability to make meaning of the circumstances and events that form the environment of relationships. Riegel's Dialectical[2] theory, that we are all in a dialogue with others in life, proposes that without empathy there is no way to know yourself in relation to others; or to give others the experience that you know them.

Imagine why co-parenting with an Asperger Syndrome mate can be such a challenge for an NT. How is an NT parent supposed to share the multi-dimensional work of parenting with a spouse who has no concept of the empathic glue that holds the parent/child relationship (and the parent/parent relationship) together?

Hopefully the answer to this question is illustrated in this book. I have written *Out of Mind - Out of Sight* primarily for the NT member of the parenting dyad; however, I expect AS parents and even adult children of Aspies to find benefit in this read. Aspies from around the world have sent me emails regarding my first book, *Going Over the Edge?* These readers say that the book has provided them with important perspective on their NT partner or spouse. One AS husband wrote me the following very powerful e-mail (I have excerpted parts.):

> *I guess your heart probably sinks just a little when you get a message from an AS man. However, I've just read your book and I'd like to thank you for its honesty and indeed bravery.*

> *I've been with my NT partner . . . for 25 years and have inflicted many distressing incidents on her similar to those you describe. But I can honestly say that none of them were ever designed to hurt. This feeling has probably made things much worse [for her]! I doubt I would have become so angry and defensive if I didn't believe myself to*

---

2 Dialectical Psychology was first introduced by Klaus Riegel. It is the only theory of psychology that comes close to explaining the AS/NT relationship since it focuses on the concept that human beings are defined by their relationships. The term "dialectical" refers to this relationship or the ongoing dialogue between people.

be 'innocent' of the crime of intention. Hopefully I am coming to re-alise that I need to do more than just not intend to do harm. . .

. . . Reading your book I think I see parallels here between my fear of being overwhelmed in social or conflict situations. But I also see similarities to those feelings when my partner expresses her frustrations and needs - to admit to her point of view seems sometimes like I would be 'destroyed.' I mention this because I get the strong feeling that you equate spirituality and loving relationships. I feel that between myself and . . . there is something very important to us both, beyond companionship. For me there seems to have been a chance given that I would never believed I would have had. . .

. . . Recently we have come to the position where we both acknowledge that possibly a split might be the only answer for us. . . In my own literal AS way, I don't think there is much I would not do for . . . if that need was not clouded by the conflict and resentment. I really hope we don't split up.

I hope this makes some sort of sense.

Many thanks once again,

T.

I hope this man's sentiments hold true for other Aspies who want to improve their marriage and co-parenting skills. As far as I am concerned, the key to success is finding a way to communicate loving intent even if the art of empathy is out of mind for Aspies.

Summary of what's to come

This book has four parts. In the first three chapters I introduce you to the daily life of AS/NT co-parenting. Like the start of any roller coaster ride, the first few hills are thrilling and gut-wrenching, but they are only a taste of what is to come. In "Helicopter Mother," "Not-So-Ordinary Moments," and "What's an NT Dad Supposed to Do?" you meet NTs and Aspies in the context of their lives—as they live them. There is no analysis, just raw emotional experience.

By the second part of the book you have a feel for the ride. You think that nothing will surprise you, but you secretly hope there is more—and there is. Be prepared to shed your preconceived notions as I introduce you to the science behind these troubling relationships. Because I believe that knowledge is power, I spend three chapters delivering the state of the art theories on Asperger Syndrome. After reading the chapters, "Empathy Imbalance," "Out of Brain - Out of Mind," and "The Rules of Engagement," your entire view of these AS/NT relationships will have changed.

With this new perspective you will have a way to experience the next four chapters with more wisdom. Instead of just responding emotionally to dramatic anecdotes, you can read between the lines. You will find yourself generating solutions for the people in these and following chapters, because you now have the tools. Be prepared to take notes.

While reading "Hapa Aspie," "Bullied or Bully," "Are You Invisible?" and "Can You Teach Love?," you ride the roller coaster toward the end of the book. You're filled with satisfaction and hope for change in your AS/NT parenting partnership.

Like any exciting roller coaster ride there is a little surprise at the end. In the fourth part of the book, I decided on more than the traditional summary and conclusion. I provide a chapter with some specific parenting techniques to help you implement the changes you want and need to make. Consider the chapter, "The Power of Intention," as a short version of the parenting manual you wish you'd had when you started your AS/NT family journey.

Part One

Chapter One, "Helicopter Mother." Without hesitation I plunge the reader into my world, the world of being an NT mother of an AS child. I'm not just a psychologist who has professional expertise on the subject of parenting with a partner who has Asperger Syndrome. I parented an Aspie child, and that has changed my life profoundly. Can you imagine what it is like for a psychologist to be clueless about AS when she discovers it in her own family? I had my master's degree in social work and my doctoral degree in psychology long before the AS diagnosis became official in the United States. My daughter was born eight years before anyone could have diagnosed her with Asperger Syndrome. By the time Bianca was officially diagnosed, at age 14, I had been a helicopter mother for years. In this chapter you will learn if you are a helicopter mother (or helicopter father) and what can you do about it.

Chapter Two, "Not-So-Ordinary Moments." While "Helicopter Mother" is an intense and painful exploration of how one AS child and one NT mother learn about each other, this chapter is about all the small stuff that creates emotional knots in AS/NT families. When you live with Aspies, it is the seemingly ordinary things that grind life to a halt. Ordinary things, such as getting enough sleep; or asking your spouse to pick up a child from soccer practice; or having a little family chitchat at the dining table. When co-parenting with an Aspie, these kinds of things can strain relationships and quickly turn into not-so-ordinary moments. Nothing you say or do works. Interaction over the simplest of things can turn unnerving and tense. And that can leave you too drained to engage fully in life.

I reintroduce you to Helen, Grant and their children, who were in my first book, *Going Over the Edge?* Helen learns how to build in stress relief for these "not-so-ordinary moments." Follow this and other families as well as mine while you learn to take back your life and create a healthier parenting style.

Chapter Three, "What's an NT Dad Supposed to Do?" When the NT parent is the dad, the parenting paradigm shifts to another dimension. These fathers, like their female NT counterparts, long for affection and meaningful communication with their Aspie spouse. As with NT moms, NT dads are startled by the inability of their AS spouse to nurture their children. Often these men are in the dark as to what is going on, because they are dealing with an undiagnosed spouse. (Aspie women are vastly under-diagnosed.) But their reaction is the same as that of many an NT mom. The NT dads are angry and hurt. They see their wives as neglectful of and abusive to their children. It feels much worse for the dads since they expect women to be the more nurturing parent. This chapter takes a look at how to resolve the gender-specific problems of being an NT dad married to an Aspie mom.

Part Two

Chapter Four, "Empathy Imbalance." In the first three chapters you were introduced to the personal experiences of some parents struggling within an AS/NT family. Starting with this chapter on Adam Smith's "Empathy = Imbalance Hypothesis" of autism,[3] the next three chapters diverge from anecdotal reports. They provide you with a theoretical foundation. Empathy has long been a controversial subject in the field of AS/NT relationships. Not only is it tough for Aspies to

---

3   Smith, Adam. "The Empathy Imbalance Hypothesis of Autism: A Theoretical Approach to Cognitive and Emotional Empathy in Autistic Development," *Psychological Record* (2009), 489-510.

INTRODUCTION: YOU ARE NOT ALONE

ascertain the minds of others and to empathize, but they frequently struggle to understand their own inner workings. Smith's research takes Baron-Cohen's "theory of mind" a step further. Through the "Empathy Imbalance Hypothesis" of autism we come to understand why so many Aspies seem to be deeply moved by life experiences and yet are unable to relate well to others.

Chapter Five, "Out of Brain - Out of Mind." Slowly Helen and NTs like her are coming to understand how their Asperger Syndrome loved ones think. But Helen also wants to know WHY her Aspies act the way they do. NTs repeatedly ask, "Why can't she SEE what I am saying?" Or they ask, "Why can't he CONNECT with my feelings?" It is not hard to see the pattern in these "why" questions. NTs repeatedly try to bring together a mutually satisfying solution. It's the one-sided, unempathic model their Aspie loved one prefers that gets in the way.

Helen got some answers to her questions when she learned about Smith's "Empathy Imbalance Hypothesis," described in Chapter Four, but she still wants to know WHY she and her AS spouse can't connect. In this chapter you are introduced to the latest neuroscience research discussed in Baron-Cohen's exciting new book, *The Science of Evil: On Empathy and the Origins of Evil*.[4] He describes a more complex spectrum of inter-connecting empathy circuits. Through the lives of the people in this chapter—Adrienne and Stefan, Jeremy and Lorri-Jane, Joe and Katrina, Marilyn and Eddie, and Marvin—you learn why Aspies struggle with empathy and connection.

Chapter Six, "The Rules of Engagement." In this third chapter on theory, I introduce the reader to *context blindness*[5] because it is important to first understand the parts of the mind/brain that are integral to

4   Baron-Cohen, Simon. (2011). *The Science of Evil: On Empathy and the Origins of Evil*. New York: Basic Books, Inc.

5   Vermeulen, Peter. (2009). *Autism as Context Blindness*. Translated from the Dutch, *Autisme als contextblindheid*. Shawnee Mission, Kansas: Autism Asperger Publishing Company.

how the mind creates meaning from context. Concepts proposed by Smith and Baron-Cohen are: cognitive empathy, emotional empathy, theory of mind, the spectrum of empathy, empathy circuits, and zero degrees of empathy. All are part of the holographic array of empathy systems that help us to create meaning from context. It is the skillful use of context that can make or break a relationship. Those who have social radar create *true empathy*. Those with empathy disorders create chaotic and sometimes destructive meaning from the context.

Celebrated family therapist Virginia Satir (a pioneer in the development of family therapy) describes parenting as "people making."[6] This brings me to one more theory that I describe in this chapter, Dialectical Psychology. [7] It wraps all of the other theories together into a cohesive context of why people-making, or parenting, is so important to a child's development. Please don't worry about the academic sound of all this. My goal is to help you use these theories in a practical way with your Aspie loved ones. Thus I have liberally sprinkled the chapter with examples from real life. I suggest one way to accommodate the problem of *context blindness* is to teach the Rules of Engagement, a template for how to relate without *true empathy*.

Part Three

Chapter Seven, "Hapa Aspie." Parenting children in a home with an Aspie parent is very complex, particularly if you have both Aspie and NT children. In the first three chapters, I described the chaos of these families, and the ensuing distress that NTs feel in this environment. In the second three chapters I outlined theories to help you better understand why Aspies do what they do. I demonstrated how to change the negative outcome by using the Rules of Engagement. In the

---

6   Satir, Virginia (1972). People Making. Out of print.
7   Riegel, Klaus. (1979). *Foundations of Dialectical Psychology*. New York: Academic Pr

next four chapters, I delve into answering specific questions about how to resolve more complex and unique parenting problems. We do need more than the Rules of Engagement to address these problems.

When interacting with a context-blind Aspie partner, the context-sensitive NT spouse has to switch back and forth between the worlds of his or her Aspie partner, Aspie children and NT children. NT children also need to keep switching. Their world is a very confusing mix. At school or with friends, they can engage in NT dialogue and reasoning that reinforces their perception of reality. But at home, they get mixed signals. As hard as it is for adults to maneuver the unusual world of Aspie/NT family life, consider how hard this is for NT children. In Chapter Seven, I discuss how NT children respond to these mixed signals. Often they develop an odd mixture of NT and AS traits that I call, "Hapa Aspie." It's a term I derived from the Hawaiian slang word, "hapa," meaning half. In this chapter, you learn how two Hapa Aspies, (Helen's son, Jason, and I) work to keep our self esteem intact.

Chapter Eight, "Bullied or Bully." Many parents of AS children have grieved over the bullying their child receives at the hands of other children. In fact, many AS adults tell me that it took them decades to heal from this type of abuse and develop a modicum of self-respect. Think about the child who is a daily target on the playground. Children can be cruel. But there is another side to the bullying that is often overlooked unless you observe an AS/NT family. Those with AS engage in bullying, too. It is often directed only at those in their home; hence when NT adults or children complain about abuse in their home, they often are not believed. Until empathy disorders, the symptoms of mind blindness, context blindness and zero degrees of empathy are understood, it is very difficult for outsiders to comprehend the chaos and abuse of which Aspies are capable. In this chapter we see how the Rules of Engagement can be applied to help Aspies regulate their emotional outbursts.

Chapter Nine, "Are You Invisible?" One very striking result of growing up Hapa Aspie is to develop a sense of psychological invisibility. I have heard many NT partners complain of this phenomenon, too. What they mean by invisibility is that they feel ignored, unappreciated, and unloved. That's because their context-blind Aspie family members are so poor at empathic reciprocity. As we have learned, we come to know ourselves in relation to others. This doesn't just apply when children are developing self-esteem. Throughout our lifespan, we continue to weave and re-weave the context of our lives, based on the interactions we have with our friends, coworkers, neighbors and loved ones.

This is why it is so important for an NT parent/partner to get feedback from their spouse. A smile, a hug, a kind word, a note of encouragement: These are messages that reinforce the NT's self-esteem and contribute to a healthy reciprocity in the relationship. Without these daily reminders from their loved ones, NTs can develop some odd defense mechanisms. One is to become psychologically invisible to others and even to themselves. In this chapter, the NT spouse learns how to take back his or her life and stop being invisible to others. This knowledge may help you help your children avoid feeling invisible, too.

Chapter Ten, "Can You Teach Love?" This question from Helen brings up the most important element in parenting—the art of loving your child, so that he or she grows up confident with a strong sense of self. But what does Helen do when her AS daughter, Jasmine, tells her mother that she isn't sure what love is? In this chapter you learn that a basic human experience, such as giving and receiving love, is not so easy when raising children in AS/NT families. Love is more than feeling it (i.e. emotional empathy). Love is more than talking about it (i.e. cognitive empathy). Love is more than systemizing a moral code to live by (as many Aspies do to compensate for their empathy disorder). Love is more than practicing the Rules of Engagement (although politeness helps).

The answer to Helen's question is worth exploring in a real and deep and heartfelt way. In this chapter, we move beyond the theories and science of empathy and social learning to see how Helen, Vivian and Todd, Anne Marie and Tony work through the dilemmas of teaching and experiencing love with their children and each other. This is the most profound work a parent can do.

Part Four

Chapter Eleven, "The Power of Intention." In Chapter Six, I introduced you to the rules of engagement where Dialectical Psychology was the foundation. In this chapter, I help you understand how to expand these rules in order to understand the intent of your AS/NT parenting partner. I show you how to express your good intentions in creative and healthy ways. These examples are not meant to be an exhaustive parenting manual. Rather, they demonstrate the power of intention. You'll see that when your intent comes from a loving heart and an open mind, communicating transcends verbal interaction. The verbal part is where so many AS/NT couples get locked down.

Chapter Twelve, "Conclusion: A New Agenda." Too many AS/NT couples and families struggle to the point of the family falling apart, because they have no help to unravel the mystery of the strange dialectic of Asperger/neurotypical relationships. By this last chapter, I hope you've learned that you are not alone, and that there is hope.

I hope that your ride on the roller coaster of *Out of Mind - Out of Sight* stirs up more than grief over the lost years with your loved ones. I hope that you are inspired to create a new agenda for parenting with your AS spouse/partner. I hope this agenda includes being true to yourself, speaking out about what you believe in, and protecting yourself and your children from abuse. Most of all, I hope your new agenda helps you find creative ways to express loving intentions no matter what the level of context blindness in your family.

Now enough standing in line! It's time to climb aboard the roller coaster and see where the ride takes us. I know the ride will be thrilling. I also hope you find it inspirational.

CHAPTER ONE

Helicopter Mother

Telling some of my own story seems the best way to start this book on parenting with a partner who has Asperger Syndrome (AS). Since authoring, "*Going Over the Edge? Life with a Partner or Spouse with Asperger Syndrome*" in 2009, I've received hundreds of questions and comments from around the world. I've been asked frequently if my ex-husband, Howard, has Asperger Syndrome. I've also been asked about my experience parenting my Asperger daughter, Bianca. Because of this interest, I'm sharing a bit of my own story.

To set the record straight, Howard never has been diagnosed with Asperger Syndrome (to my knowledge). It would be improper for me to even speculate about this. Bianca, my spirited and spritely daughter, was diagnosed with Asperger Syndrome by three different mental health professionals and a school psychologist when she was 14.

I'm not just a psychologist who has professional expertise on the subject of parenting with a partner who has Asperger Syndrome. I have parented an Aspie child, and that has changed my life profoundly.

Can you imagine what it is like for a psychologist to be clueless about AS when she discovers it in her own family? I had my master's degree in social work and my doctoral degree in psychology long before the AS diagnosis became official in the United States. My daughter was born eight years before anyone could have diagnosed her with Asperger Syndrome. By the time Bianca was officially diagnosed at age 14, I had been a "helicopter mother" for years. (I still am to some extent even though Bianca is 26 and has left home.) You know the type don't you? She's always hovering over her very dependent child.

I visited countless professionals, read dozens of books, and scoured the Internet for information on Asperger Syndrome. I had Bianca try vitamin/mineral supplements, special diets, psychiatric medications, sensory integration therapy[8], psychotherapy, and brain scans. I enrolled Bianca in private specialty schools and Internet schools. I homeschooled her and hired tutors. You name it, I tried it, all in search of answers to the growing social/emotional/intellectual/health problems my daughter was experiencing as she approached adolescence.

In this chapter, I highlight my more memorable experiences with Bianca. I offer them not from the perspective of the professional expert, but from the experience of a mother on a journey into the world of her child. Like the parents I write about in this book, I was taken by surprise with my daughter's problems. I had no special knowledge to help her, just a mother's love. I had to learn from the "outside in" and change many of my basic beliefs about parenting in order to reach her. I made some profoundly moving discoveries along the way. I made some terrible, life-altering mistakes, too.

My story diverges slightly from the theme of this book, because I cannot personally speak to co-parenting with an Aspie. I can, however,

---

8   Many people with ASD are over-sensitive or under-sensitive to sights, sounds, temperature, touch and so on. As a result of these sensory sensitivities, they can benefit from a type of occupational therapy defined as "sensory integration," which is designed to reduce their over and under reactivity.

describe first-hand the depressing, painful, fascinating and joyful journey of parenting in a family of Aspies and neurotypicals (NTs). Judging from the overwhelmingly supportive responses I've received from around the world regarding my first book, *Going Over the Edge? Life with a Partner or Spouse with Asperger Syndrome,* my perspective is right on target for those NT moms and dads who are co-parenting with an Aspie partner or spouse.

The Oklahoma prairie

In a dimly lit motel room, I sit in front of my laptop, uploading photos from the day's exploration on the Oklahoma prairie. Next to me, sprawling on her bed, is my 15-year-old daughter, Bianca. She's reading a novel, her usual pastime. She is re-reading *Raptor Red*. She loves this book so much, and reads it so often, that she's literally worn it out. I have bought her more than one copy to keep her happy.

Raptor Red, a book about dinosaurs, is a very fitting choice since we are participating in a field trip sponsored by the Paleontological Society and the University of Oklahoma. By day we sight dinosaur tracks permanently etched into rock where millions of years ago a mighty river dried up and created mud flats, the perfect medium for storing ancient footprints. On another day, we follow our guides past fences and "No Trespassing" signs to witness evidence of dinosaur nests with bits of fossilized eggshell still scattered on the ground. Amazing. I take most of the photos, because Bianca is mesmerized by the experience. She needs the photos to document the field trip for school credit. As usual, I remain the "responsible party," a trait of helicopter mothers the world over.

Bianca is the youngest member of the expedition and kind of an honorary member since most participants are professional paleontologists, graduate students, or adults with an amateur's passion. In true helicopter mother fashion, I'd searched high and low for a way to leverage my daughter's interest in paleontology and art into a high school science credit. I had to be inventive in those days since there were no educational programs for "twice exceptional" kids at the time (i.e. Asperger Syndrome and gifted).

In 2001, I'd made a call to Dr. Jere Lipps, paleontology professor at the University of California at Berkeley. Lipps had been very gracious. He'd told me that Bianca was more than welcome to attend the North American Paleontology (NAP) Conference to be held at the university that summer. (I still have the NAPC coffee mug.) Bianca was only 14 then and received an award for being the youngest participant. I was very proud of her—even though she'd needed a dose of Klonopin (an anti-anxiety drug) to make it through each day.

But we aren't in Berkeley tonight. We are out in the middle of nowhere on the prairie, in a forlorn sixties-type motel. I am uploading pictures from the camera, picking out the best shots and inserting them into a PowerPoint presentation. It is Bianca's task to write a description of each photo. That will be a test of her paleontological knowledge as well as a test of her limited patience. She complains that she is tired. She complains that she is hungry. She complains that she can't remember anything. She complains about me and my helicoptering. With enough coaxing and bribes of snacks from the hotel canteen machines, Bianca finishes the PowerPoint for that day. We celebrate by calling Dad and her sister, Phoebe, to say, "Good night." Then we fall into bed exhausted. I sleep well, knowing my daughter is a day closer to earning that science credit.

All told, Bianca and I attended three NAP conferences. Can you believe it? She was able to work with the leaders in the field! She has their autographs. She attended the premier of "Jurassic Park" in Bozeman, Montana. The hosts were the famous paleontologists who'd contributed not only their professional expertise but their personalities to the film; the main characters were fashioned after real paleontologists. A couple of these researchers even offered to mentor Bianca through her science projects since her high school required an "expert" to approve her work in order to get school credit.

It's not easy being a helicopter mother, but it would have been harder yet to watch my child fail in school. I found all kinds of ways to work around the school system. I hired tutors to coax her through Spanish. I negotiated high school credit for art through Portland's Pacific Northwest College of Art. For physical education credit, I logged Bianca's hours on the treadmill in the basement.

After losing several tutors to Bianca's outrageous tantrums, I finally found a retired college professor who was not threatened by her moods. He stuck with her for two years, thank goodness. (He also was invaluable when we needed him to mediate between a frustrated teacher and my eccentric child.) When Bianca became eligible to take classes at the local community college (as a gifted 16 year old), I felt a huge burden leave my shoulders. She was entranced by history and women's studies courses. Although I still had to coax her through the homework and draft many of the outlines for her papers, Bianca passed all exams on her own. She is smart if not disciplined.

The fanciful little girl

It wasn't always this challenging. When Bianca was a preschooler, she was delightful and charming. I have wonderful memories of both my little girls. One in particular is the balloon episode. Bianca and Phoebe had been chasing a balloon in the backyard. Every time they'd try to catch the balloon it would waft out of reach, and they'd burst out giggling. I have a picture of them wrestling with the balloon. They look so cute. They were carefree little girls then, sisters as I'd hoped they would be.

I remember when 3-year-old Bianca helped Daddy make a video at Yellowstone National Park. She'd used a toy plastic moose and pretended it was foraging through the trees. She'd made great sound effects! Daddy had been proud of himself, too.

I can still hear Bianca's beautiful little-girl voice singing the songs she learned in pre-school. She had a marvelous memory, and music was her forte. Somehow songs always soothed her. One of my favorites from that precious time is "Big Bugs:"

> *"Big bugs. Smawl bugs.*
> *Big bugs. Smawl bugs.*
> *See dem cwawl.*
> *On da wawl.*
> *Keepy, keepy cwawling.*
> *Nevah, nevah fawling.*
> *Bugs, bugs, bugs.*
> *Bugs, bugs, bugs."*

Bianca always loved books of course. What self-respecting hyperlexic[9] Asperger child doesn't? She acquired words at an amazing rate and taught herself to read by the age of 4. (In fact I used to embarrass Bianca when she got older by showing the photo I took of her reading one of Daddy's legal advance sheets while she was sitting on the potty!) By the end of kindergarten, Bianca was considered an "independent" reader. By the end of first grade, she was reading at sixth-grade level. Bianca took a book with her everywhere we went. One time she even read on the raft as we dodged rapids on the wild Salmon River in Idaho: She had promised to put the book in her life vest and grab the safety rope if I told her that a tough rapid was coming up! I adored her for loving books and took great pride in introducing her to reading. But it wasn't my influence that made her love reading: It was Asperger Syndrome.

---

9 Hyperlexic means an extraordinary ability to decode words. With regard to autistic children, this usually equates to early reading and even teaching oneself to read.

I'd wondered a little bit about Bianca's social skills by the end of first grade. She never seemed to play with the other children and actually shunned them if they got too rambunctious. I dismissed my concerns and chalked it up to her sensitive, fanciful spirit. She loved to play "pretend" all by herself. She wrapped herself in colorful silk scarves from her toy chest and would dance and sing in her room—all alone. She was charming and guileless, my fanciful little girl.

Bianca's amazing and unusual attention to visual detail was a constant surprise to me. As a 5 year old, she got the teacher's attention when she drew a picture for a Christmas card she'd created. All of the children were instructed to draw pictures that represented Christmas to them. There were delightful and childish drawings from Bianca's classmates—Christmas trees, candy canes and Santa Clauses. But Bianca's was the most intriguing. She'd drawn a Nativity scene, and baby Jesus was drawn anatomically correct! Ignoring the tiny penis on Baby Jesus, I'd asked why she'd chosen a Nativity scene for her subject. She'd said, in a rather matter of fact manner, "The teacher told us to draw what Christmas represents." Her teacher and I had laughed, but I'd wondered, even then, if Bianca was smart, or just too literal.

Bianca continued to develop her art through drawing. She had no patience for any medium but pencils and crayons, even as she got older. Her drawings were phenomenal. She drew on every scrap of paper she could find, even restaurant napkins if Mommy forgot a drawing pad. One day when she was about 7, I asked her what she was drawing. She explained that it was a drawing of Mommy. Indeed I could see the resemblance, down to my characteristic earrings, red lipstick and smile. I was flattered and held up the picture to inspect it. As I turned the paper in my hand, I noticed a disturbing drawing on the other side. Before I could ask, Bianca said, "That's Daddy. He's frowning. He always frowns." I knew she was right about her daddy, but I didn't know what troubled him.

The "wonder years"

The "wonder years" are supposed to be the time from about age 6 to age 10 or 11. This is the time when, generally, children are enthusiastically exploring their newfound independence. Their curiosity expands beyond the family yet they are still delightfully innocent. Although they are cultivating friends and acquiring social and academic knowledge at school, they really do still adore their parents. As you will learn in following chapters, this is also the period of time when children are learning about social context. In other words, they are developing a theory of mind that is a prerequisite for empathy. Empathy leads to a whole host of social skills required in the worlds of children and adults. Bianca's "wonder years" were anything but typical.

At the end of first grade, and about the time other children had made their first best friend, my daughter asked me if she could leave private school and attend public school, so she could ride the school bus. She had no friends to ask over to our house, so she wouldn't miss them if she moved to a new school. Bianca was problem solving in the systematic and logical way that Aspie children do. Bianca must have realized that she didn't fit in at her private Montessori school, although her teachers were all very kind. She reasoned that she might do better at public school if she could ride the bus and meet new children. Logical.

I don't know why I acquiesced to Bianca's request, but I did. Perhaps I'd hoped that Bianca was right and that she would finally make friends. The following year she started second grade at the public school. I have lots of regrets about this now. Bianca was no more accepted in public school than she was in private school, and she actually was protected less. She became fearful of riding the school bus, because of the taunts of other children. I started driving her to school again.

One day as I drove Bianca home from school, I looked in the rearview mirror at my precious daughter and attempted a conversation. She was now using her big-girl car seat, with her younger sister in the little-girl car seat. In spite of myself, I asked the question uttered by many a parent on the drive home from school, "So Bianca how was school today?"

No response from Bianca, who appeared to be daydreaming out the window.

"Bianca?" I pressed. "Honey, Mommy's asking you a question. I was just wondering what you did in school today. Tell me about your day please." I smiled in the rearview mirror, hoping she could see that I was speaking to her. I couldn't tell if she was looking in the mirror or spacing out.

Still no response.

I turned on the radio and listened to the music for a moment. But I didn't want to give up, so I turned it off. Aren't mommies and daughters supposed to chat once in awhile? So I tried again with a bit more desperation in my voice. "Bianca, sweetie? Would you mind chatting with Mommy for a moment? I really want to know how school is going for you since you are now in second grade."

Bianca appeared to move her head in my direction ever so slowly. Her pupils were wide and black as if she was being called back from an hallucinogenic experience. She pondered my question for a few seconds before giving me a careful and even response. "I'm thinking," she said.

I was encouraged. Oh yes she finally heard me. It must be noisy in the car. She's just like her daddy, I thought to myself. I often have to prompt him a few times before he responds to me. My own mother, an Aspie, was the same way. I remember as a child sometimes getting so desperate for my mother to pay attention to me that I would call out her given name rather than the characteristic, "Mommy." With renewed hope that I might have a sweet conversation with my little girl, I asked her enthusiastically, "Oh and what are you thinking about?" I was smiling broadly with fervent anticipation that we might connect, Mommy to daughter/daughter to Mommy.

"I'm just thinking," Bianca said with that same even tone. Then she turned and looked out the window. Sadly, I got her message. Bianca was silent for the rest of the trip home. I turned the radio back on.

I have lots of memories like this of Bianca from age 6 to 11. This is when I'd started to get desperate. Throughout the "wonder years," I became a classic helicopter mother. I registered Bianca for Brownies, soccer and piano lessons. I sent her to summer camps for the arts. I forced her to audition for a prestigious private choir because of her marvelous singing ability—even though she was frightened of the other choir members. I tried everything I could think of to search out activities that would make my autistic child smile. I moved her back to a small private school. During these years my office manager and I created a color-coded calendar to coordinate the transportation efforts of five adults in service to my two children. Yes five!

Bianca was always miserable in group activities and thrived only on the attention of adults. She was picked on at school. When I asked for help, the teachers and administrators thought I was over-reacting. Bianca wasn't complaining about her social isolation, so they reasoned I was an irrational helicopter mother. No teacher, school counselor or school administrator ever suggested that Bianca might be autistic. The term "autistic" didn't surface until years later. I discovered the diagnosis myself, during my desperate search to help my gifted daughter.

It was during the "wonder years" that I consulted a naturopath for the first time: Bianca's pediatrician was at a loss as to what to do. My Aspie mom had been very conscientious about what I ate as a child. Similarly, I'd created an organic, pesticide-free diet for my family. In spite of the healthy diet, Bianca always had a rash or a runny nose.

Her body was so sensitive that when she came down with chicken pox (There was no vaccine at that time.), she had lesions over her entire body, even between her toes and inside her nose. Poor thing.[10]

When Bianca entered puberty at age 11 she started to experience extreme moodiness that would last for days, sometimes for two weeks. At the onset of her menses, Bianca's premenstrual Syndrome (PMS) was so devastating that she would vomit. I could predict the start of her PMS each month by the phone call I would get from the school nurse. The naturopath was extremely helpful, but Bianca's special diet turned our lives upside down: no sugar, no gluten, no corn, no dairy, no fruit! I adapted, and Bianca got a bit better. She even recognized the benefits. One day as I dished out the supplements the naturopath had prescribed, Bianca said to me, "You know Mom, our family is lucky that I have all of these allergies, because we can all eat better." I was happy that she'd accepted her special needs and didn't feel deprived.

Middle school meltdown

I made another terrible mistake when Bianca was 13. I removed her from her third private school and sent her off to the public middle school for eighth grade. She was failing at the private school, and she was tormented by the other children. Furthermore, the eighth-grade teacher there bullied her. (Fortunately he was fired the year after Bianca left the school.) So I took a chance and placed her in the Talented and Gifted program at the local middle school.

The middle school teacher was an experienced professional, who assured me that she had taught many students like Bianca. Those assurances fell by the wayside within six weeks. After a short period of complaining

---

10 Many people with ASD have a variety of immunodeficiency illnesses such as gluten and dairy intolerance. My daughter is even intolerant of most fruit. It is not surprising that those with ASD also seem to suffer more severely from childhood illnesses, such as chicken pox or ear infections.

about Bianca, the teacher decided the better approach was to ignore her for the rest of the year. Clearly Bianca was still an outsider, an oddball, a victim. By the end of middle school, Bianca had straight "F" grades. Howard stepped up and negotiated a "peace treaty" with the school. They agreed to let her "pass" eighth grade as long as we didn't ask for more (such as a special needs assessment and special education services). How very convenient for everyone, but still no diagnosis and no help.

Bianca made a valiant effort to participate in the social world of middle school. One day she brought home a fund-raising kit from school that included the usual magazine subscriptions so many schools use to raise supplemental income. Instead of just leaving the flyer for me to peruse, Bianca asked me to subscribe to "Teen" and "Cosmo Girl." I was stunned. She had never shown any interest in makeup or fashion. To further my amazement, she asked to go shopping for some makeup. I was thrilled at sharing this special mother/daughter experience. I still remember the day we went to our local shopping center to buy eye shadow. I'd asked her what colors she would like. She'd said, "Oh I don't care. You pick it out." That should have been a clue.

After two months of receiving "Teen" and "Cosmo Girl," Bianca told me to discontinue her subscriptions. She said, "I don't think the girls at my school are like the girls in these magazines. They don't help me." I was speechless! It was then I realized that Bianca was trying to fathom the social world at school by doing research on the subject. It was similar to her notion in first grade that riding the school bus to public school might bring her some friends. I was depressed. I kept hoping Bianca would learn to adjust and fit in the way other children do. It was becoming obvious that was not to be. My heart was breaking for her lonely attempts to fit in.

It was during this time that Bianca's mental health had begun to seriously deteriorate. Her emotional meltdowns were so severe that I decided to consult psychiatrists. She would cry and scream and threaten for hours. She cursed her tutors and threw books at them. She began mutilating herself by digging huge holes in her skin and scalp. She cut off chunks of her beautiful hair and hid the hair in her dresser. She became frightened of insects. She hoarded food in her room. She saved odd bits of lint and fuzz, rolling them into little balls and storing them in a decorative box. I was terrified. I felt all alone to help my precious child. When I consulted my husband, he offered no ideas. His solution was to work more hours and be away from home more. This was the beginning of the end of our marriage.

Being the supreme helicopter mother that I am, I'd rolled up my sleeves and started calling local psychiatrists and psychologists. After a few appointments, it was clear these local folks weren't going to be much help. I got on the Internet and began searching for help outside our community. I found physician Daniel Amen, who was then promoting his work with ADHD.[11] I liked his philosophy: Understanding mental illness requires looking at the brain, not just at behavior. I made an appointment immediately, and our whole family flew to Dr. Amen's Newport Beach, California, clinic for two days of evaluation and SPECT scans (i.e. single photon emitted, computed tomography).[12]

Ever alert to an opportunity for Bianca to get some school credit, I took photos of the experience, which Bianca later used in a PowerPoint presentation for her eighth grade culmination project. Amen determined that Bianca had ADHD and anxiety.[13] To address these issues, he

---

11   ADHD or Attention Deficit Hyperactivity Disorder is commonly known as ADD. The major symptoms are hyperactivity, distractibility. It is most often first noticed in childhood, because of problems in the classroom.

12   Dr. Daniel Amen pioneered the use of SPECT scans, a type of brain scan. In his research he has discovered patterns in brain scans that help to diagnose ADHD and other brain disorders.

13   To his credit Dr. Amen has researched more about the autism spectrum since he first met Bianca. At the time however, he did not recognize the pattern that is so evident in Bianca's SPECT scans.

prescribed Adderall and Paxil for Bianca. I was hopeful. The medicine did help for awhile—a little while.

Of doctors, drugs and divorce

Bianca was terrified to return to public school after the horrific experience in eighth grade, so more research by the helicopter mom. This time I found Willoway, a private Internet academy. It boasted a unique educational community. It had a virtual campus complete with avatars for students and faculty. Bianca loved it. Between Willoway and a private tutor, she managed to secure substantial credits by the end of ninth grade. She didn't have to deal with people much, just avatars. She could hide in her room and emerge only briefly for the few family demands made of her.

Emotionally though, Bianca still suffered. In high school, Bianca's art began to show more distress. Dinosaurs and fairies were replaced by gaunt figures in tattered clothing. Frequently her human characters had spears piercing their chests, blood dripping to the ground. She told me, "But they can't die Mom because they are vampires. They can only suffer." I knew this morbid thinking wasn't good. By this time, Bianca was taking a cocktail of psychotropic medications, including Adderall, Paxil, and Risperdal (an anti-psychotic medication). She was considerably overweight, too, even on the organic, whole food diet.

> This time I found a private Internet academy. . . . It boasted a uniqe educational community. It had a virtual campus complete with avatars for students and faculty. Bianca loved it. . . . She didn't have to deal with people much, just avatars.

Her doctors couldn't break through to help her even though we now had the diagnosis of

Asperger Syndrome. It was a nightmare, and I felt more helpless than I ever had.

About the time I'd stumbled into the possibility of Asperger Syndrome, Bianca had had a premonition. It came in the form of a story she wrote for a history class at Willoway. I continue to be amazed at the minds of autistics. If we NTs can step aside from our notions of how communication should work, we might hear what autistics are trying to tell us. They use a different language. Poetry and music and other arts often provide a window into their souls. I know this is true of Bianca.

Bianca's assignment for her study of the Roman Empire was to write a fictionalized diary of a person who lived in ancient Pompeii before the great volcanic eruption that buried the city. Bianca chose to write about the life of a Roman girl close to her own age of 14. Bianca cleverly wrote the date and time of each entry, as if the girl were actually writing a daily diary. The girl described living with her mother and father in a lovely Roman house with servants. She described Father as a hard-working sort of guy, who paid little attention to his wife and daughter. Mother was very concerned about the frightening volcanic activity at the mountain and begged Father to let the family leave Pompeii. Mother talked to others in the village about her concerns: Each day she and her daughter watched their friends leave the city and flee to safety. But Father was firm and dismissed Mother's complaints as idle gossip.

Then, on a day when Father was away, Mother, Daughter and a male servant made their getaway. Mother had been planning this for some time. She knew that the volcano would blow any day, and she'd decided to leave with or without her husband. The three of them made it to the boat dock before Father discovered them. He was angry and menacing. He snatched the girl from her mother's arms and told Mother that she could leave—but not with his daughter. As he carried the girl away from her mother and into the danger of the volcano, Bianca had written:

> *He just grabbed me and walked away. I tried to fight him and get back to Mother but he just flung me over his shoulder. I could hear Mother wailing, "I love you Little One! I love you," and sobbing her heart out. I sobbed too. The sound of this day will stay with me forever; the sound of the calling of the sea, my mother's wails, and my father's stubborn silence.*

Bianca ends the diary with the eruption of Mt. Vesuvius. The girl is home alone in the garden when it erupts, abandoned by her father who finally ran away, too. As volcanic rocks and ash rain down, the young Roman girl writes her last entry in the diary:

> *I know I am going to die. But in the face of death there is no fear, remorse or guilt. Only a tired kind of grief I could not be with my mother as the mountain fulfilled her prophecy. I doubt this journal is going to last this disaster but just in case, Mother if you find this pleas . . . .*

Bianca was prophetic. Within five months of the fictional diary's creation, I'd filed for divorce from Howard. It is certainly a common, but sad, story that so many AS/NT marriages end in divorce (symbolized in the diary by Mother leaving on the boat). Even today, with better diagnosis and treatment available for children with Asperger Syndrome, at the end of the day parents still have to go home to a difficult situation (demonstrated by the pending eruption of the volcano). Aspie children still have to live with the pain of being different, dreadfully different, from the norm (represented by sitting in the garden alone). These very dependent children also fear separation from their primary nurturing parent (shown when Father takes the daughter from Mother in Bianca's story). Furthermore, their NT siblings grow up feeling like Mom and

Dad, so focused on the AS child or children, don't have much energy left for them. It is a very lonely existence for everyone.

The aftermath of Vesuvius

I would like to tell you things got better for Bianca and all of us, but just like in her Pompeii diary, our lives turned tragic. Howard and I divorced. It was extremely hostile as I described in my first book on Asperger Syndrome. Bianca continued to deteriorate under the pressures of divorce. There were times when she would throw herself to the floor, screaming and writhing with intense emotional pain. One time she ran outside as I was leaving for an appointment and threw herself in front of my car. Sometimes she would stand outside my home office door and scream at the top of her lungs. My office manager could not contain an 18 year old with such rage, so I would have to excuse myself from my client(s) and try to comfort Bianca. Human beings are remarkably resilient, or I wouldn't even be writing this book: I have survived the tragedy even if I grieve daily.

Just about the time I'd thought I could take no more, there was another volcanic upheaval. Bianca left for a two-week summer visit with her father in August 2005. She was 18. We had just returned from Kauai where I had taken the girls to celebrate Bianca's graduation from high school. During that visit, and unbeknownst to me, Howard and his new wife had gone to Europe and left Bianca in the care of a house sitter. I received a fax from Howard after he left, informing me that he was out of the country, unreachable and wanted no contact from me. When I went to his house to bring Bianca home, the house sitter called the police. The police told me that I was trespassing. I left without my daughter and went home, terrified for my daughter's safety while alone with a stranger. I sobbed myself to sleep. It was all just as Bianca had predicted in her story of the girl in Pompeii—separated from her mother and abandoned by her father.

I didn't know it at the time, but this would be one of the last times I'd see Bianca. She never returned from her father's house. My phone number was blocked at Howard's home, so I was unable to call her there. Bianca's cell phone was disconnected. In eight years, she's never responded to my emails or letters. I tried seeking her out at the community college where I learned she was taking classes, but she complained to campus security that I was dangerous and crazy. The officer asked me to leave the campus. I received one letter from Bianca when she was first gone. It said that she was disavowing me as her mother forever.

I used to cry myself to sleep each and every night. The anguish over losing my daughter was too unbearable to describe. My fears for her safety skyrocketed after she was taken from me. How can a helicopter mother protect her child if the child is gone forever? Many years later I came across a police report from that time period. It revealed one thing that had happened with Bianca. (It was as if the mother in Bianca's story of Pompeii had finally found her daughter's diary.)

The incident that brought the police to Howard's house had happened shortly after his return from the European trip and coincided with the letter of denunciation Bianca had sent me in October 2005. Paradoxically it is comforting to know more about what happened then, because it's less of a mystery now. The pain survives, but more of the puzzle has come together for me. Apparently, Bianca had been in full meltdown mode at Howard's house during and after that summer visit. Howard had called the police, because he'd thought Bianca was suicidal. The responding officer had noted in his report that Bianca had stashed knives all over the house and was threatening to use them. Howard, frightened, had wanted Bianca taken to the hospital. By the time the officer had arrived, Bianca's condition had stabilized: She'd apparently taken some medication to calm down. The officer had written that Bianca has "ashburger's disorder."

What's my story have to do with you?

My goal in writing this brief summary of my life with Bianca is not to frighten you, but to give you another perspective on the life of one NT trying to co-parent an AS child. Nor is this chapter meant to address all of the AS/NT issues. It is just a sample of my life. Raising ASD and NT children with an ASD spouse is probably the most difficult and complex job you will ever do. I am confident that my story is not so different from those of you reading this book. Yes, there are many stories just as extreme, and I will tell some of them in the succeeding chapters.

Being a helicopter mother (or a helicopter father) is a natural outcome of the crazy-making AS/NT world we find ourselves in. Our natural instincts are to protectively hover over our children when they have such a serious disability. It is equally natural to fight for them even if neighbors, teachers, and authority figures deem you unreasonable.

You can probably see a myriad of mistakes that I made in parenting Bianca. For one, I was in denial for a very long time. Perhaps if I had found a knowledgeable psychologist sooner, it would have ended differently. Perhaps the divorce could have been avoided had Howard and I been helped to work together better. Perhaps Bianca wouldn't have suffered so much if she had been diagnosed earlier. Perhaps if she had been born 20 years later, she would have had a few more resources to help her cope.

There are serious drawbacks to helicoptering, too. It leaves you very little time to relax and enjoy your children. Because, as the super-responsible parent, you are always in survival mode. Bianca used to say of me, "My mom is obsessed with my brain!" Sadly, she was not equally aware of my love for her. That is my fault as a helicopter mother. I'd circled her with offers of help while not leaving enough time for hugs.

Thank goodness there have been improvements in understanding Asperger Syndrome in the last decade. We certainly have a long way to go to help our AS/NT families. I believe this book is a start in the right direction. If we hope to save the Biancas of the world (and their parents from a lifetime of grieving) we must have the courage to look at the harsh realities threatening our families I hope this book brings you healing just as writing it has for me. To paraphrase what my beautiful, special daughter Bianca wrote in her Pompeii diary:

> *I don't know if this book will ever reach you but just in case,*
> *Bianca,*

> *If you find this please . . . forgive me. I will love you forever.*

Lessons learned

1. Helicoptering is a natural by-product of loving your very dependent child. Don't let anyone tell you that you are over-reacting. Your strongest asset is your heart.

2. Channel your helicoptering into finding a good psychologist or Asperger Syndrome specialist, who really knows what he or she is doing. Then you don't have

to helicopter so much. Nowadays there are many more and better-trained professionals to help you.

3. Join a support group for NTs in relationships with Aspies. I sponsor an international group online at www.meetup.com. It's called Asperger Syndrome: Partners & Family of Adults with ASD. Find us at http://www.meetup.com/Asperger-Syndrome-Partners-Family-of-Adults-with-ASD

4. Read everything about Asperger Syndrome you can get your hands on. There are marvelously supportive resources at Autism Asperger Publishing Company. See http://www.aapcpublishing.net/

5. Join your local Autism Society affiliate. It is important that you socialize with other parents and spouses who share your experience. You are not alone. There are others who have gone before you and can help you avoid the pitfalls of ignorance. You'll find a list of these groups at http://www.autismsource.org/

6. Don't blame yourself for your mistakes. This is a challenging walk. You are bound to be positively transformed by your Aspie(s) just as I have been. Remember, you're also apt to make some terrible life-altering decisions. Love yourself enough to keep on creating a meaningful life in spite of your mistakes. Keep in mind that human beings are remarkably resilient.

7. Take time to relax and play. The future is unwritten, but today is a gift to be relished with your loved ones.

CHAPTER TWO

Not-so-ordinary Moments

While "Helicopter Mother" is an intense and painful exploration of how one Asperger Syndrome (AS) child and neurotypical (NT) mother learn about each other, this chapter is about all of the small stuff that creates emotional knots in these families. When you live with Aspies, it is the ordinary things that cause life to grind to a halt. Ordinary things, such as: getting enough sleep; asking your spouse to pick up a child from soccer practice; or having a little family chitchat at the dining table.

Everyone else takes these ordinary things for granted. They don't give them a second thought, because life just flows. This means that they have time to attend to more rewarding things in life. An NT parent trusts that an NT partner can: remember things; follow through with things; take care of him or herself, and demonstrate respect. But when co-parenting with an Aspie, these ordinary things become strained and turn into not-so-ordinary moments. It feels as if you are Alice in *Alice's Adventures in Wonderland*, attending the tea-party with the Mad Hatter and the sleeping Dormouse. Nothing makes sense. Nothing you say or do works. Even doing something simple is unnerving and tense, leaving you too drained to engage more fully in life.

I reintroduce you to Helen (an NT), Grant (an AS) and their children from my first book, *Going Over the Edge?* The children are Jasmine, who is an Aspie and Jason, an NT. Here, Helen learns how to build in stress relief for those not-so-ordinary moments. You'll follow this family and others, and share my personal experiences, as you learn to take back your life and create a healthier parenting style.

Dinner is for sleeping

The following story was related to me by Helen at one of our psychotherapy sessions. She often gets so involved in the story that it feels as if you are sharing the drama with her. I have not changed Helen's words in the retelling since it is the way in which Helen tells the story that reveals so much about AS/NT relationships.

Helen recounts what happened when Grant fell asleep at the dinner table.

Grant's head gradually slid to his chest as he dozed off at the dinner table. He was still holding his fork with that peculiar grip of his, using the fork like a soup ladle with his little finger sticking straight out to the side. Grant has an unusual way of doing a lot of things. This is not the first time he has fallen asleep at the dinner table while poised for another bite.

I didn't notice him falling asleep at first. He often sits with his face close to the plate, shoveling in his food with his "ladle." I suppose that is why he has spots on his tie and food drippings on his shirt and pants. A meal with the family is not important to Grant for the social value. It is a time to eat and nothing more. Well, occasionally it is apparently also a time to nap.

I have seen Grant fall asleep in a restaurant when we are out to dinner with friends. Usually he doesn't snore, thank goodness. I suppose that is because he falls asleep sitting up. Of course I am embarrassed by these moments and hope no one notices that Grant has fallen asleep. I gently nudge him, hoping that he will quickly recognize the social faux pas and quietly resume his comportment. Nope. Not Grant. He wakes up with a startle and screams loudly, 'What's the matter?' He looks at me as if, by waking him, I have done something terribly wrong. By then the jig is up, and the whole restaurant snickers. I am mortified.

This time we are home, all seated around the dinner table in the kitchen. I didn't notice Grant fall asleep right away, because my 15-year old twins were being so cute. For a change they were laughing and enjoying each other. I was having fun, too. We don't often laugh together. Jasmine was teasing Jason a bit about his soccer uniform. The colors really are atrocious, so bad that even Jasmine actually noticed. Jason got her back though. He told her that her boobs jiggle when she eats. I flinched when he said this, thinking Jasmine would get hurt or mad and fly into a rage. Instead, she laughed an uproarious laugh and made her boobs jiggle even more!

It was the laughter that woke Grant. I noticed him wake with a startle. The fork fell from his hand and hit the plate with a clatter. The sound made him startle even more: He usually has no awareness of where he is when he awakens. It's like he is in this deep coma when he falls asleep. Maybe he drifts off to another universe at these times. When he wakes up abruptly like this, he is confused, angry and shaking all over. He slammed his hand on the table and yelled, 'Enough! Stop your laughing. Settle down and eat your meal.'

He stared daggers at the children, so they tried to comply. But they were deep into giggling and jiggling and just couldn't suppress their merriment. *You know how it is when you are a kid. When you try to stifle a laugh, the laugh just comes spitting out of your mouth and your nose. Jason was spit-giggling so violently that a piece of lettuce shot out of his nose! Then Jasmine just fell apart with laughter, and so did I. Grant only got more furious. 'Enough!' he said as he pounded his fist on the table again.*

'Grant, honestly, it's okay,' I said between chuckles. 'The kids are just having fun. Now guys settle down a bit, and eat your dinner please.' I tried to support Grant, even though tears of laughter were streaming down my face. He is their father and an authority figure. But I also wanted the children to know that their transgression wasn't all that bad.

Grant got even more furious. 'The dinner table is no place for laughing. It's dinnertime. It's time for eating and nothing more,' he said adamantly. We all fell silent this time under the spell of his stern pronouncement.

I looked at Jason and Jasmine. A slight smile crept over Jason's face as he looked at the twinkle in my eyes—and at his sister's newly developing 'boobs.' We both wanted to say it, but we dared not. We wanted to say, 'Yes Dad. The dinner table is no place for laughing. Only for eating—and sleeping!' A little snicker snuck out in spite of myself.

On the other hand, Jasmine was sitting there looking confused and hurt, and probably blaming herself. I had to do something. I couldn't leave her there all upset about what was going on. She doesn't understand the nuances of the moment like her brother and I do. So I decided to confront Grant, even though a meltdown was imminent. Or maybe it was to fend off a meltdown from at least one of my Aspies.

'Grant honey,' I said, 'I know we startled you, but you did fall asleep at the table. Maybe you didn't notice, but you did.' I tried to use a gentle tone, so he wouldn't take offense. I looked at Grant's face and waited for any sign of acknowledgment. There was none, so I continued, hoping he was tracking. It's hard for him to track when he gets this upset. 'Besides,'

I said, 'dinner is also a time to socialize. Sure it's a time for eating, but also a time for conversation. We are such a busy family that we don't always get a chance to catch up with each other. It's fun to share dinner, chat about the day and even laugh a bit. I know the kids may laugh at silly kid things . . . but then they are kids. Relax a bit and enjoy the moment.'

I could tell that Grant wasn't buying any of it. He didn't argue with me, thank goodness, but he sat there in stony silence. So did the rest of us. No more laughing. I had a lump in my throat from the last bite I had taken. I couldn't swallow it. Maybe that is why I have gastric reflux. You know what gastric reflux is don't you? It's where food gets stuck in your esophagus and hurts so badly that it feels like you are going to explode. Sometimes I have to vomit to take the pain away, because the food is just stuck, stuck. Caused by one too many 'Grant' moments at the dinner table, I guess.

I looked at the kids. I could tell they were 'done,' so I let them leave the table. 'Don't worry guys. I'll clean up. Just go do your homework. I'll come check on you later and see if you need any help,' I said to the kids. I avoided Grant's gaze in hopes that he was 'done,' too.

There was silence the rest of the evening.

Take R & R to stay well

I could feel my own esophagus tightening as Helen wove her story of dinner with her family. With all of those stress chemicals hurtling through her body on a daily basis, it is a wonder that she

> Consider these breaks R & R from the war zone. Military organizations recognize the need for R & R for soldiers always under the pressure of hyper vigilance. Why not the NT parent?

has her health at all. Many NT spouses/partners report a variety of psychosomatic and immunodeficiency illnesses, such as migraines, arthritis, gastric reflux, and fibromyalgia. Even weight gain occurs as a result of the hypervigilance required to parent with an Aspie. When the body is regularly thrown into a state of alarm, the over-production of adrenalin and cortisol wreaks havoc with the body's natural defense mechanisms. These alarm systems are designed for short-term emergencies, not for the daily crises regimen common to NT parents married to Aspies. Left unchecked, real physical illness can emerge in NT parents.

I advise Helen often that she needs to take care of her physical health, even more so than other people. Regular massages, long walks with friends, Yoga, a swim, or workouts at the gym are rejuvenating and healing after draining episodes such as the one at the dinner table. Consider these breaks R & R from the war zone. Military organizations recognize the need for R & R for soldiers always under the pressure of hyper vigilance. Why not the NT parent?

With R & R and proper nutrition, Helen can make better decisions for her children, even when Grant is clueless. There is no doubt that Jasmine already suffers severe anxiety because of her Asperger Syndrome. She is anxious most of the time, poor kid. Helen is always in protective mode around Jasmine. But what about Jason? He is torn between his parents on a regular basis. He walks on eggshells around Grant and his sister most of the time. Just about the time he starts to relax and have some normal family fun, a not-so-ordinary moment occurs. Then all of those stress chemicals flood his system, too. Jasmine gets her mother's attention and protection during these incidents. Jason gets sent to his room to do his homework.

Helen can't be all things to all people. She is living in a war zone along with her children. Survival comes first at times like these. Jasmine is fragile, so her mother reaches out to her first. Helen needs to find another way to parent her children instead of tiptoeing around Grant. That sends the children mixed messages.

One good thing going for Jason is soccer. Helen started him in the sport when he was only 5. He not only loves the game and is a pretty good athlete, but he gets a chance to be with other families that handle life very differently than what he experiences at home. Helen is grateful for Jason's soccer coach, a loving family man who views the camaraderie of teammates as important as skill training. Through soccer Jason gets a physical release for those stress chemicals. And, he gets to experience a loving, child-centered, adult male role model.

Sleep problems and the small stuff that steals quality parenting time

In the above story, Helen revealed a lot about the small stuff that erodes her ability to parent effectively. Grant's mind-blindness, or the inability to know what is going on in the minds of his wife and children, creates the kind of rigidity that leads to the no-laughing-at-the-dinner-table rule. There is also the strong possibility that Grant has a sleep disorder. Otherwise, why fall asleep during the social hour of a family dinner? Helen also references Grant's odd eating posture—head to chest while gripping his fork like a shovel, his little finger extended. Those with Asperger Syndrome often acquire odd body postures or movements. This is a compensation for poor motor control and/or for never having learned the social graces. All of these things are wearing for an NT parent who is raising children and trying to keep the household running efficiently.

Helen continues with another example of exhausting not-so-ordinary moments.

You know Dr. Marshack, I used to think Grant's oddities were cute. He was kind of childlike and charming. I had no idea when we first met and fell in love that his not-so-ordinary everyday behaviors could be such a drain on my energy. If it were just the two of us, I think I could endure it, but with the children, I keep feeling like a rotten parent. I am always covering for him and protecting the kids and trying to find just a little moment of sanity for us to have fun. But all of Grant's rigid behaviors keep getting in the way.

Like this one time when I was filming a spot on a television talk show. As a family practice naturopath, I was asked to talk on some health subject. I can't even remember it anymore, but I remember how Grant handled [the situation]. It was so embarrassing.

The show was being taped in the evening at about 7, but would air during the day. This is one of those talk shows where you take questions from the audience, kind of like 'Oprah.' Only it's a local show. I should be so lucky! Anyway the producer told me that it was okay to bring my friends and family to the taping of the show, even the children. She wanted to introduce my family to make the show more family friendly and helpful to young families. I think the twins were about 4 at the time. So I invited a few people and told them to dress casual, but nice-day casual. You know what I mean.

I had to be at the studio early, so I told Grant to bring the children later. I knew they would be staying up late, but with good naps I'd hoped they could handle the nighttime event. Oh my goodness you won't believe what Grant did. He is just so clueless. I can live with this faux pas and the kids weren't harmed, but gosh he can be dull! Do you wanna know what he did? Of course I did. I nodded my head and sat on the edge of my seat waiting for her punch line.

Well, there he was in the audience with the kids all smiles. But the kids were dressed in their sleepers. It's a daytime show, and my screwball husband brings the kids in their sleepers for all the world to see. [It made me look like] some nutball professional mother who doesn't know how to dress her kids for the day. At least Grant wasn't wearing his jammies!

Helen had a wry smirk on her face. She was frustrated with her husband but willing to laugh it off.

Helen continues describing her reaction to Grant bringing the children to the taping of a television show in their pajamas.

I still have the tape from that show. Ugh! But what was worse was trying to explain the problem to Grant. He gets so uptight that he cannot accept any criticism. He just kept telling me that he'd wanted the kids ready for bed when they got home. He just got stuck there, like the food in my throat. He is always so worried about making sure the kids get to bed on time that he couldn't put that aside for one day to help me with my career. He couldn't see what was wrong with having the kids in their sleepers for a daytime television show! But you know he thinks laughing at the dinner table is wrong. Things are always okay for Grant if they are his idea and wrong if they are our ideas. More of that mind-blindness as you call it.

Sometimes I feel like screaming over these things, but I know they are small stuff. You know the expression, 'Don't sweat the small stuff.' But what do you do when your life is turned upside down every day by the small stuff? How can I be there for my twins when I am always upset with their father? What kind of example am I setting of the way married people should be?

Sweat some of the small stuff

Yes it is the small stuff of the day that interferes when co-parenting with an AS spouse. It is pointless to tell an NT parent not to sweat the small stuff when it is the small stuff that is the problem. All of those small-stuff events that turn into not-so-ordinary moments are taxing. The NT parent knows all too well that ignoring the small stuff can lead to dire consequences. But you just can't stretch yourself that thin.

The key to success in parenting, any parenting, is to attend to those things you can and let the others go. In Helen's case, beating herself up for being a rotten parent is no help. She needs to be there for herself, her children and her husband as she can. Even if family members suffer under the constraints of an NT/Aspie family lifestyle, the suffering is less if you take off the unnecessary layer of self-recrimination. Your children need to adjust to the family they have and learn to make the most of their lives. It is good mental health to face life realistically and with a positive attitude even if you can't do it all.

A sleep problem is one of the small things that shouldn't be ignored. Notice that Grant is overly concerned about the children being ready for bed. Do you suppose that has anything to do with his own anxiety about the children's nighttime bed ritual . . . or his own sleep disorder? Many Aspies have sleep disorders but the cause, the etiology, is unclear. There is so much still to be discovered about these physiological problems. Jasmine, for example, seems to run on a 25-hour clock. She isn't just off by an hour. Each day she is off by another hour and yet another hour, so that eventually her day turns upside down. Helen has reported finding her daughter wide awake at 2 a.m., entertaining herself with reading or the Internet—clearly not getting the rest she will need for the next day in school.

Another possibility with the sleep problem is diet. Grant refuses to listen to Helen's suggestions about a healthier diet. There are staunch supporters of a gluten free, dairy free, and sugar free diet for those on the autism spectrum. The idea is that food allergies cause stress for the body, which in turn leads to fatigue and eventually auto-immune illnesses. Grant, on the other hand, prefers to buy lunch at a mini-mart or fast food restaurant. He skips breakfast altogether, because he is too tired in the morning to eat. With this poor nutrition, is it any wonder Grant is worn out by dinnertime, falling asleep at the table much like a drunk who's been on a bender?

A number of my clients have reported this phenomenon with their Aspies. Without the normal sleep cycle of going in and out of deep sleep to lighter sleep and so forth, it is possible that Aspies are not really getting a good rest. We need sleep cycling to rejuvenate our bodies. If Aspies are just falling into a dead sleep, they may awake as if from a hangover instead of refreshed. It is possible that these anomalies in sleep patterns rob Aspies of a good night's rest and poise them to have increased anxiety over everyday things.

Detach from those not-so-ordinary moments

Parenting in your AS/NT family requires caring for yourself first. In the chaos of family life, it may seem impossible to create time for you. It is possible if you learn the art of detachment. Detachment is learning to protect yourself from all of those not-so-ordinary moments. Stop taking it all personally. Stop worrying if you've covered all the bases. Stop beating yourself up for your parenting flaws. Stop expecting more from your AS spouse than he or she can deliver.

When you learn the art of detaching, you actually free up some energy to care for yourself. And that creates the energy to make better decisions instead of flitting from crisis to crisis. Detaching helps you psychologically step back and allow others to solve problems for themselves. Ultimately, isn't that what all parents want—for their children to become independent, self-sufficient and able to enter the adult world "ready to roll?"

There are two methods for achieving detachment. One is emotional self-care, and the other is cognitive self-care. Emotional self-care is doing all of the feel-good things you can fit into your day. Of course they should be healthy "feel goods." If you notice that you are drinking or eating or smoking too much, you need healthier self-care. Make it a point to always plan healing rest and recreation in your day. I know it is a lot to ask when you are juggling so much, but if you don't take care of yourself, who will take care of the family? Attend to the priorities you must, and drop the rest. If you don't, you'll wind up ill. If you wind up ill, there will be more to drop. Avoid the vicious cycle of failure and depression.

Some simple "take-a-break" ideas are walking the dog, getting a manicure, calling a friend, doing some deep breathing and Yoga stretches.

Cognitive self-care consists of education. One major cause of stress is lack of information. When you can't fathom what is going on with your Aspie, and they are accusing you of things you didn't do, stress increases exponentially. It is bad enough to be misunderstood. It is quite another to have no frame of reference for the misunderstanding. Even though it is work to read a book and to attend psychotherapy, knowledge is power. Clear up the mystery around your Aspie's thinking and behavior by educating yourself about autism and Asperger Syndrome. When you understand that those with Asperger Syndrome are more tuned in to the facts and the "truth" than they are to your feelings, it is much easier to manage a conversation. It still takes more time and energy than an NT/NT conversation would, but this knowledge provides a base from which to solve the problem. Cognitive self-care helps you to detach and to feel less emotionally drained.

Lessons learned

1. Don't let anyone make you feel badly about sweating the small stuff. If they do not live with a co-parent who has Asperger Syndrome, they have no idea that it is all small stuff.

2. Because your Aspie co-parent gets hung up on the small stuff, it can grow to many not-so-ordinary moments. While you may not be able to stop this progression, at least you can take the mystery out of the process: Learn about Asperger Syndrome. Don't take things so personally: This is the NT's version of "don't sweat the small stuff."

3. Always and every day take R & R breaks for yourself. Without this necessary rejuvenation, you will get sick.

4. Stop beating yourself up. You are being the best parent possible in a tough situation. Your kids will gain more self-respect and personal strength if they learn to tackle life as it comes.

5. Spit-giggle, "jiggle" and wear your jammies more often. Since you are going to be out of sync with the rest of the world anyway, you might as well enjoy it.

CHAPTER THREE

What's an NT Dad Supposed to Do?

When the neurotypical (NT) parent is the dad, the parenting paradigm shifts. NT dads are just as startled as NT moms are by the inability of the Asperger Syndrome (AS) partner to nurture their children. Often these men are in the dark, because they are dealing with an undiagnosed spouse. (Aspie women are vastly under-diagnosed.) Their reaction is the same as many an NT mom's: They're angry and hurt. NT dads see their wives as neglectful of and abusive to their children. Since women are expected to be the more nurturing parent, these feelings are magnified for an NT dad. Without help, the NT father gets angrier and angrier. This clouds the real problem—his undiagnosed Asperger's wife and her limited parenting skills.

The parents of Devin are a good example. Neither parent is socially polished. Both are high school graduates and successful at modest careers. When Devin was diagnosed with Asperger Syndrome by his elementary school psychologist many years ago, neither parent really sought help. They never read a book, or attended a support group, or sought out psychotherapy. Instead, they left Devin's welfare in the hands of the school district, which provided minimal special education services. With each year that passed, this NT father got angrier and angrier and blamed his Aspie wife for being a neglectful mother. Ultimately the marriage failed, and Dad watched in anguish as his son also failed.

Let's take a look at how to resolve problems that arise when an NT dad and an Aspie mom are trying to rear children together. Could Devin's family have made it if Dad had availed himself of psychotherapy and education earlier on? Would Dad have become so locked into his anger if he had? Could the entire family have benefitted from education on the rules of engagement for an AS/NT family? (I will be talking about this in our next three chapters.)

The boy who likes snakes

This is my first meeting with Devin, a pleasant-looking boy of 12. He is the youngest child of two, and his parents are divorced after 20 years of marriage. Devin was diagnosed with Asperger Syndrome many years before but has had no treatment and not much in the way of academic support. Although Devin is well-behaved, his mother is worried that he seems immature socially and unprepared for the demands of middle school and high school. Actually, a close friend is the worried one and encouraged Mom to seek professional guidance. Devin's mom had struggled to define the problem when I'd met with her the week before. I knew that she was concerned about Devin's grades. So, while Mom looks on, I start Devin's first session with the subject of grades to get the conversation going.

"Hi Devin. I'm Dr. Marshack, but you can call me Kathy if you wish." Devin smiles weakly at me but says nothing.

I continue, "So Devin, you know, your mom brought you here today, because she wants some help for you in school. Were you aware of your mom's concerns?"

Devin doesn't look at his mom for any encouragement. Instead he examines my face very carefully as if looking for clues to the answer. After a few seconds, he says, "No."

"Well okay then." This is not an infrequent beginning with some of the more introverted AS children I treat. Typically, they sit politely and wait for me to ask questions. They form a response, but there is no real conversation. I decide to try another tactic with Devin. "Tell me Devin, what do you want to be when you grow up?"

Devin doesn't move a muscle, but this subject gets his attention. "I want to be a reptile biologist," he says, sitting very still. There is no sparkle in his eyes even at the mention of a subject he cares about. He doesn't look for approval from his mother. He doesn't send those signals that NTs send to indicate they want to engage in conversation about a favorite subject. But reptiles seem like a hot topic for Devin, so I decide to pursue it.

I hung in there. "Oh, reptile biologist? So is there any one reptile you are especially interested in?"

"Snakes." Devin immediately answers. Moving the pace up a bit he adds, "I like snakes."

Devin's mother makes no sound. She sits there as still as her son. I wonder if Mom needs me to give her permission to join the conversation. I turn to her, smile and say, "What do you think of Devin's interest in snakes?"

With the same characteristic slowness of speech and non-committal smile that I see on Devin's face, she says, "Yes, he always has been interested in snakes." Then Mom turns her head away from me and looks in Devin's direction. She seems to be waiting patiently for my next question.

Things are going slowly, but the subject of snakes is my faint hope to open up communication. "So Devin, you like snakes and want to be a herpetologist?" As I ask, I nod my head to encourage his interest in talking.

Devin says, "Yes, that's the word for reptile biologist. I didn't think you would know the word, so I didn't say it. But yes, I want to be a herpetologist. I have handled snakes, lots of snakes."

Wow! That's a lot of talking. My hope increases that I have finally found a subject to provide me entry into this young man's life. "Oh my! You have handled lots of snakes? You must have pet snakes then. (I take an unwarranted guess.) Do you have an aquarium or something like that for your snakes?" I look hopefully at Mom and Devin. In typical NT fashion, I've jumped on the subject and am trying to push it along, so that we all can "relate."

No response from Mom, but Devin says, "No."

I'm puzzled and look to Mom for help. She weakly offers an explanation that makes no more sense than Devin's story. She says, "We don't have snakes in the house, but maybe he handled them at his dad's house. You know he lives out a ways in the country, so maybe that is where Devin handled them." (I later learned that Dad lives about five miles from me, hardly a rural area. We have few snakes in western Washington State. Mostly we have garter snakes, those harmless, uninteresting reptiles that eat bugs in the garden.)

Devin waits while his mother and I talk. I try to confirm Mom's notion about snakes at Dad's house. I turn to Devin and say, "Could that be where you handled the snakes, at Dad's house?"

"No." Once again Devin cannot help me out. He is locked into his black-and-white-world where he waits for my next question.

"Okay then. So you don't have a snake aquarium, and you haven't handled snakes at Dad's, so maybe you have handled snakes in Mom's backyard. Could that be it?" Perhaps I smiled outwardly with my discovery that Devin may have "handled" garter snakes in his backyard. I know I was smiling on the inside.

"Yes," he says.

Ah ha! My AS radar has finally kicked in. I ask Devin, "Lots of snakes in your backyard?" I continue to smile as I close in.

"Yes," he says.

"Hmmm," I wonder aloud. "So Devin, do your friends like snakes?" I know that Devin has no friends, according to his mother. He spends all of his time inside in front of the computer or television or playing with his older brother. But who knows if this pattern changes when he visits his father? I will discover that next week when I meet Dad for the first time.

"Yes, they have handled lots of snakes," Devin responds.

By now it is clear that Devin is not really conversing with me in the traditional sense of connecting with another person. There is no real reciprocity, no real empathy. Like so many on the autism spectrum, he has learned a few rules of engagement, but he is applying them in such a limited fashion that he gives himself away. Devin has a good intention as I will discover. I decide to see how outlandish Devin's story will get—and if his mother will engage. I wonder about her own ability to relate.

I continue. "Well Devin, so you have handled lots of snakes in the backyard is that right? And maybe you have handled snakes in your dad's backyard, maybe not?" I look in Mother's direction in a feeble attempt to draw her into the conversation, but she does not respond. I look back toward Devin and continue, "And your friends have handled lots of snakes, too?" I feel like a sales rep moving my client toward agreeing to buy a new life insurance policy. I don't really want Devin to buy anything, but talking with him is definitely like trying to convince someone to buy something they don't want.

"Yes," he says. Warming to the task at hand, he offers a major contribution to the conversation. "I have been bitten, too." Mom still doesn't budge. She doesn't look at me but stares steadfastly at Devin. Sensing that he has my attention, Devin says, "I've been bitten lots of times." I think I even see a twinkle of amusement in his eye.

Now I have him! I really want to see how far he will go, but I don't want to offend him. I just want to investigate the depth of his disability. "So Devin have your friends been bitten, too?"

He seems to be enjoying this "conversation," although he never gives me more than that weak half smile—and the twinkle. As we descend down the rabbit hole, Devin offers a response much more quickly with each question, and there is a growing tone of enthusiasm in his voice. "Yes!" he says, adding, "They have been bitten several times!"

I look at Mom and ask, "Are you aware of any of this—that Devin has been bitten by snakes?" With the same look as her son, that pleasant but non-descript half smile, she says, "No."

"Okay then," I say to Mom as I sit back in my chair. "Let me clear up what I think is going on here."

I lean forward toward Devin and gently confront his lying. I smile at him. There is no tone of recrimination in my voice. I want him to know that I am here to help him; however some things have to shift if he is to make the changes he needs in his life. "Devin, I believe that you like snakes. I believe that you want to be a herpetologist when you grow up. I believe that you have handled a garter snake or two in your backyard." I pause and watch Devin carefully. "But I doubt that you have ever been bitten by a garter snake. What do you think?"

Devin ponders my complex question a bit. Then he actually smiles as if he has a clever answer. "Well maybe they just nibbled me," he responds as he tries to recoup his losses.

"And nibbled your friends, too?" I joke with him to see if he will come around, but he doesn't. He just sits there along with his mother, waiting for my next question. Or perhaps he's realized that the jig is up, that he has finally come to the end of the line.

Looking back and forth between Devin and Mom, I explain what I believe is going on. I smile again at Devin and, from across the room, lean toward where he sits on the couch. With no disrespect for his words or his non-verbal presentation, I begin gently, "No Devin, I don't believe the snakes nibbled you either. They didn't bite you, and they didn't nibble you. But here's what I think you are trying to do. Do you want to know what I think? (He has no response of course.) I think you are trying to have a conversation with me. Since you like snakes, you can talk about that subject. So you made up some things to tell me, because you want to be polite when I ask you questions. What do you think? Is that what you were doing?"

Devin smiles back at me and says, "Yes." I hope in that moment that Devin feels his good intentions were understood and appreciated. This young man has tried for years to comprehend the complexities of human interaction. He smiles. He answers questions politely. He attempts a version of chitchat, such as fabricating tales. He obviously wants to please. What is missing is the empathy that opens the door to meaningful relating between people.

Devin and his mother live parallel lives. She never asks questions, and he never tells her what is in his mind. He has been "promoted" (advanced to the next grade level) each year at school, but his test scores show that he has acquired very little academic knowledge for a seventh grader. His school has provided a variety of special education services over the years. However, not once has Devin's Individual Education Plan (IEP)[14] included social/emotional/behavioral goals— other than very rudimentary things, such as putting his name on his

---

14   An IEP or Individual Education Plan is required by Federal law for those students who have a disability. School districts are required to conduct a special education evaluation of students with ASD and determine a plan to meet their special needs. The IEP is evaluated annually for needed changes as the student matures.

paper and turning in homework on time. Devin's father suspects Devin
has been bullied at school, but he has no proof of it. (It seems there are
never any school reports of Aspies being bullied.) That's probably because Devin keeps such a low profile at school that he is overlooked by
the staff and the students.

How Dad sees it

The next time I saw Mom by herself, I reviewed Devin's psychological evaluation and reconfirmed the Asperger Syndrome diagnosis. I
discussed with her the need to upgrade Devin's IEP, so that it includes
more comprehensive social/emotional/behavioral interventions. I
referred her to private classes where Devin could practice social skills
over the summer. I told Mom that it is very important to get intensive
help for Devin right away: He is soon to enter high school where he's
apt to fall seriously behind and be seriously miserable, because of his
immaturity and minimal social skills.

I wondered to myself why Mom had not done these things six
years before when Devin was diagnosed with Asperger Syndrome.
Perhaps professionals had tried to encourage her but weren't as direct.
She could have been waylaid by the divorce process, but that was
years ago. Why did she wait until now to finally get some help? On
the other hand, if Mom has ASD like her son, she, too, needs a more
concrete plan of action to follow. The plan needs to be spelled out in
detail. Without guidance, Mom and Devin will continue just drifting
along.

I asked Mom if Devin's father would participate in helping, too,
especially since he lives close by and has regular parenting time with
his son. Mom agreed to give Dad my phone number, but she doubted
he would cooperate. She said Dad was very hostile. She told me that
she and Dad haven't talked much since the divorce. Mom also said that

Dad doesn't believe Devin has any problems at all. Instead, Dad blames Mom for Devin's immaturity. And Mom knows he does.

The next day I got an email from Mom indicating that she had already registered Devin for the summer program for kids with AS. Plus she had contacted the school to get started developing a new, more informed IEP. I also got a call from Dad, who rearranges his schedule to meet with me in two days. I was pleased that both parents were ready to pull together for their son.

Unlike his ex-wife, Dad has lots to talk about at our session. He is anxious to get help for Devin, but it has never occurred to him to seek psychological services. He complains that his concerns were ignored by the court when, during the divorce, Mom was given physical custody of Devin. He complains that Mom is neglectful; after all—Devin never plays outside and is left alone all of the time. Apparently Dad has gone back to court several times in order to reverse the custody agreement, and he's lost more money each time. Dad even complains that Devin's older brother does all of the parenting, because his ex-wife is never home. Dad is just plain disgusted with his ex-wife. He believes she is the cause of all Devin's problems.

I can tell that Dad really cares about Devin. His lack of information about Asperger Syndrome has created his animosity more than any mistakes made by his ex-wife. Like most parents, he believes that children develop as a result of raising, training

> Human beings come into this world with a certain genetic loading that unfolds as they mature. . . . how children are "wired" has a huge impact.

and teaching them. He doesn't seem to be aware of the "nature-nurture" concept that children are influenced by both their innate traits and the parenting they receive. Human beings come into this world with a certain genetic loading that unfolds as they mature. True, this genetic makeup is influenced by parenting, schooling and the social world, but how children are "wired" has a huge impact. According to current research, how we develop is more related to our innate genetic makeup than to any parenting technique.[15] I will discuss some of these theories in later chapters.

I share the snake story with Dad, and he is speechless. He agrees it sounds like something Devin would say, but Dad clings to the "neglectful mom" theory as the cause. He believes Devin makes up things like this because he is lonely and because his ex-wife does not parent properly. Dad cannot let go of blaming Devin's mom, so I level with him.

"It's time to stop being angry with your ex-wife and start helping Devin," I say. "Mom may have made mistakes as a parent. Perhaps she isn't as attentive to Devin as you would like. But Devin is a difficult child to parent, because he has a developmental disorder. He is autistic. He isn't like other children who can learn from the social milieu. He keeps to himself, because he has found a quirky way to cope in a world that revolves around interpersonal interaction—something at which he is terrible."

Devin's dad looks at me intently, as if comprehending for the first time something very important about his child. He leans forward silently with a look that encourages me to continue. I say, "I also believe it when you tell me that Devin's older brother does a lot of the parenting. More like protecting. He may recognize that Devin is different; hence be trying to help Mom out. Obviously the anger you have toward your ex-wife makes it difficult for the children to come to you about problems they have with their mother. Your older son may step in to help with Devin in order to help Mom and to avoid confrontation

---

15   For example, research published in the British medical journal "Lancet," February 28, 2013, shows the genetic relationship between schizophrenia, bipolar disorder, ADHD and autism. These disorders were once thought to be much more related to nurture, but with the latest genetic research we realize that more of who we become is related to our genetic makeup.

with you. Can't you see how your frustrations may be making the children more protective of their mother and more unwilling to talk with you?"

Now Devin's Dad has tears of recognition in his eyes. "I know you are angry," I continue. "I realize that you have felt helpless to intervene with Devin. You've tried using the courts: See how well that worked! Now it is time to take a different approach." I'm emphatic, and it pays off. Dad softens. (I have not diagnosed his ex-wife with Asperger Syndrome. She didn't ask for that kind of help for herself.). Dad feels heard, for the first time, about his fears for his son. Then he reveals where his anger originated.

Dad's face is flushed as he holds back tears of relief. "You know Dr. Marshack, I've realized for a long time that there is autism in my family. One of my brothers has a child with Tourette's Syndrome.[16] One of my cousins has a child who is severely autistic. And then there is my son Devin. We were all talking the other day about how autism has found its way into our kids' generation, but I am not sure where it started in my family."

This is huge progress for an NT Dad who, moments before, only had anger guiding him. More than likely, this NT Dad grew up with autism in his family. He was angry and confused as a child and felt abandoned by his parents. He didn't want this for Devin. He admits that he would still be married to Devin's mother had she not filed for divorce. As unhappy as he was in the loveless marriage, he would have stayed, so that his children didn't feel abandoned. Now he is crushed to learn that years of anger have blinded him to the kind of parenting his boys need.

Devin's dad left the office with a lot to think about. He'd asked me for the names of the professional references I had given his ex-wife.

---

16 Tourette's Syndrome is related to ASD genetically. It is characterized by both motor and vocal tics.

He'd agreed to contact the school and actively participate in the IEP process, too. He'd smiled wryly as he'd told me, "I can't promise you that I will ever be able to talk to my ex-wife about all of this, but I will do whatever it takes to get help for Devin. He's a sweet kid, and I want the best for him."

I'd smiled back and said, "I know you love your son. Now it's time to put the anger aside and do the work for Devin. He's almost grown. He needs a father to show him how to be a man. I'll help you all I can."

Dad had reached out his hand to shake mine. "Thank you," he'd said as he turned to walk down the stairs. I hope healing can begin for this family.

How other NT dads handle the anger

Matt slumped down in the chair and announced, "I can't take it anymore. We've finally agreed to a divorce. Ever since our son was diagnosed with autism last year, I have read every book I could get my hands on. I have attended classes and support groups. Heck I even started a dad's group with the Autism Society. But I think I am going to have a heart attack and die if I have to live one more day with my wife. She treats our children like animals. It's not that she is angry so much as she is impatient. She can't understand their needs. How am I supposed to work to support my family, parent my autistic child and our two other children, plus clean up the damage my Asperger's wife does all day long when I am gone?"

Matt was trembling as he spoke. "I know Matt," I say. "You are a great dad, and you have worked so hard on this marriage and for your family. I am sure Marina does appreciate your devotion even if she doesn't know how to tell you."

Matt continues, "Oh I know Marina is trying, but I am just exhausted and discouraged. Marina depends on me to take care of it all ,and

I just can't anymore. When the kids are acting up, she turns invisible, or she does the exact opposite and screams. She complains that I don't understand how hard it is for her when I ask her to take care of some small thing. She uses her diagnosis as an excuse to get out of doing anything for the family. She can't cook dinner or clean because the children are too messy or too noisy, or whatever. Smells send her through the roof. Did I tell you that she left the house two nights ago just as I was cooking dinner? She said the smell made her want to vomit. Gosh, I know she is super-sensitive to smells but does that mean she should be treated like a princess?"[17]

"I'm so sorry Matt," I say. "It does sound like Marina needs more than a diagnosis. How is the therapy going with the marital therapist by the way?" (I am Matt's psychologist. His wife has another. Together they see a third therapist for marital therapy.)

"Oh yeah! That is certainly going nowhere! Our marriage therapist is always telling me to settle down, that Marina is trying, and that she needs me to help more with the children. Really? I wish the therapist could understand what I need. Marina works part-time, and now she wants to go full-time. I guess she feels more comfortable at work among adults than with our children. Our son has to have full-time care, because he is severely autistic. Who's supposed to do that? There are bills to be paid. So here's my plan."

I listen patiently as Matt explains his plan. He has decided to file for divorce and move to the basement of the family home. His reasoning is that the family cannot afford the divorce if he moves out. By living in the small quarters in the basement, Matt figures he'll gain emotional space and still be available to the children. When the children are grown, he can move out and finalize the divorce.

---

17   Among the sensory sensitivities that many with ASD experience, the sense of smell is often one. A heightened sense of smell can render a person with ASD unable to participate in a social function.

"How does Marina feel about this Matt?" I question.

Matt says, "Well of course she doesn't like it, but it is better than fighting all of the time. Plus I do want to help her, but [moving to the basement] is all that's left for me."

"Matt . . . do you still love Marina?" I know that he does even if it is a one-sided relationship.

"Of course I love her," responds Matt. "But I can't live like this. I can handle Asperger's. What I can't handle is an asshole! Marina is abusive and neglectful. It will take years of therapy for her to get better if she ever does. My kids can't wait to have a happy childhood. I want to show my children that there is another way. I think I am making a stand by moving to the basement. It may be weird for them in one way. But in another it is sending the message that it is not okay to put up with Mom's craziness. . . . .I love my wife as part of the family, but I long ago gave up seeing her as my best friend and lover. Do you know what I mean?"

Yes I do know what Matt means. He is angry because that is what men do . . . get angry when they are depressed and afraid. But nowhere in his plan is there really anything for Matt. He wants to get away from the pain of his AS/NT marriage, yet he doesn't want to abandon his family. He came up with a compromise that is unlikely to work. Will he really have some peace in the basement? Will Marina handle everything more smoothly when her husband is not on the main floor of the house? Will the kids really leave him alone when they have come to depend on him for everything? Will he succeed in making the point to the children that Mom's parenting is "craziness?" Matt has a long road ahead of him.

NT dad Raleigh found a very similar solution to his dilemma years before Matt thought about living in the basement. Raleigh's 40-year-old Asperger's child still lives with him and his wife Debbie. Raleigh and Debbie sleep in separate bedrooms and have done so for decades.

The other children are grown and left home long ago. Raleigh does not eat dinner with his wife and son. He works late hours and often on weekends, too. He might watch a little television in the family room, but he heads for his bedroom without saying goodnight to his wife. Occasionally he plays golf with a friend. Raleigh long ago gave up asking his wife to join him in socializing. Raleigh is doing his duty but lives a loveless existence.

When the NT Dad asks for help

"I have to say I am here as much for myself as for my daughter, son-in-law and baby," says Natalie, a 60-year-old NT mother and now a grandmother. Sitting next to her on the loveseat in my office is her daughter, Kendra, recently diagnosed with Asperger Syndrome by a local neuropsychologist. Across from Kendra and her mother are Kendra's husband, Jakob, and the couple's adorable 2-year-old boy, who is happy in Daddy's lap.

Natalie speaks for the family. "When I learned about Kendra's diagnosis and then researched ASD on the Internet, I felt just terrible about how I've treated Jakob and Kendra. I thought that Jakob needed to be more tolerant of Kendra, because she was a new mommy and still learning her way around motherhood. I told Kendra that she needed to be patient with the baby and to try harder . . . as if that would work. I feel just terrible being the meddling mother-in-law, but I was just trying to help. Now that I realize my daughter has Asperger Syndrome, I understand the anguish that Jakob feels and how depressed my daughter is. Can you help us Dr. Marshack?"

Emboldened by Natalie's support Jakob picks up the dialogue. "It has been six long years of frustration and anguish over just what's wrong. When Kendra got diagnosed everything just fell into place in my mind. I finally had an answer to my questions about her. I am so

OUT OF MIND - OUT OF SIGHT

grateful that my wife decided to follow up with a diagnosis." Jakob smiles lovingly at Kendra, and she smiles back. "And if it weren't for Natalie, we wouldn't have come so far in such a short time." Natalie and Jakob exchange looks of appreciation.

"But," says Jakob, "my first priority is our son, Mathias." Jakob goes right to the heart of the matter. Kendra's diagnosis is a big help, but it isn't therapy. She needs a lot of tools. I need a lot of tools. We all need a lot of help to make it as a family. Mathias is only 2 years old, and I am terrified that Kendra's mind blindness and lack of empathy will cause him irreparable harm. Now don't get me wrong. I love my wife, and I know she is willing to commit to whatever it takes. Right Honey?" Kendra nods her head in agreement and continues to let her husband speak for both of them.

Natalie shoots a look of reassurance at Jakob as he continues. "It's just that I can already see the signs of verbal abuse and impatience. I really hate complaining like this, but we want some help." Jakob asks plaintively, "Can you help?" Jakob, Natalie and Kendra had all read my book *Going Over the Edge?* and had agreed that nearly every chapter hit close to home. Now they are ready to take the next step and learn how to parent together. Jakob is worried since nothing seems to break Kendra out of her Aspie ways.

Because the couple's babysitter, grandma Natalie, is at our first session, I'm able to witness firsthand some of the problems that Jakob bemoaned. The precocious little boy keeps going over to Daddy for interaction. When the toddler spies the candy bowl in the waiting room, he asks repeatedly for candy. I provide toys, but he wants Daddy's attention. . . and candy! The child is adorable, and I assure the parents that I don't mind the inconvenience. I suggest that we do our best to work around Mathias. As Kendra's tensions grow, she roughly grabs a toy from her son's hand. Natalie quickly picks up the toddler to protect him from his mother. She passes Mathias to Jakob when the toddler reaches for his Daddy. Natalie makes a short apology and offers to take Mathias out of the room, so that the couple can continue to talk with me. I suggest that both Jakob and Natalie take Mathias into the lobby for a few minutes while I talk with Kendra alone. This will give Kendra some breathing room to allow her anxiety to settle down.

After the door shuts, Kendra says, "Thank you," with a sigh of relief. "I really get unnerved by Mathias' constant badgering for stuff. I know I should be more patient, but he drives me crazy."

I say, "Well most parents of toddlers lose their patience once in awhile. It takes time to learn how to handle it." I'm trying to be encouraging, but Kendra has another intention.

"No it's not that. I am selfish," Kendra comments quite candidly. "I really cannot tolerate the noise at all. I want him to shut up most of the time. I know this isn't good for him, but it is just the way it is. Sounds, smells, lights . . . .I'm just too sensitive and can't stand it when Mathias whines. Jakob is really the better parent. Do you hear any voices coming from the lobby? The fact that it is quiet out there tells you that Jakob knows how to relate to Mathias. Mathias just likes him better."

A few moments later Kendra proves her point. I ask her to exchange places with Jakob, so that I might chat with him alone. The noise level grows in the lobby as Mathias begs his mother for candy and can't seem to be comforted at all by her. I hear Natalie trying to soothe both of them. Then I hear the door slam as Kendra leaves the office. Later we learn that Kendra had decided the stress level was too high. She'd gone outside, lit up a cigarette and paced back and forth by the car while Natalie watched Mathias inside.

Turning over the entire job of parenting to Jakob is not the answer. Neither is co-parenting when Kendra has so little tolerance for normal toddler behavior. Natalie is a backup only rarely since she is still actively engaged in her career as a high school teacher. This couple will have to find a method for co-parenting that's different than those touted in the standard "how to parent" books. At least this couple is starting early to develop a parenting plan that meets the unique needs of an AS/NT family. Hopefully, they can design a structure that gives Mathias all of the love and support he needs to grow up with a healthy self image. Hopefully, Jakob and Kendra can stay in love with each other for years to come. Hopefully, Kendra can learn more positive methods for regulating her emotions. Hopefully, Jakob can find, in Kendra, the helpmate he needs. Then, hopefully, Jakob won't feel so alone in his worries about Mathias.

Lessons learned

1. Anger and withdrawal are common ways NT dads deal with parenting problems associated with marriage to an Aspie wife.

2. NT dads should recognize the anger for what it is, depression. They feel trapped by the double bind of wanting to protect their children and wanting to be free of the emotional neglect in their marriage.

3. Even in our contemporary society, the role reversal for NT dads is hard. Each must adjust to an Aspie partner who lacks empathy for her children. That's tough when motherhood is so highly revered.

4. Get professional help. Trust that your anger is not without reason. Know that staying angry will make you sick and destroy the family.

5. It is advisable to find your own personal therapist, separate from your marital therapist. NT dads need a safe place to talk and resolve their feelings of anger without being destructive.

6. Divorce may happen but court is no place to resolve the Asperger's in your family. If you have to opt for parallel parenting (parenting in two homes), at least be educated about ASD.

7. It is not surprising that many NT dads grew up in families with members who were autistic. These men may unconsciously have sought out an Aspie spouse, because it is a dynamic with which they are familiar.

8. Nature versus nurture is the long-standing theory that children are influenced by both their genetic makeup and the social/emotional environment in which they grow up. When parenting with an Aspie mom, an NT dad faces a nature versus nurture dilemma.

CHAPTER FOUR

Empathy Imbalance

In the first three chapters you were introduced to some parents struggling within Asperger Syndrome (AS)/neurotypical (NT) families. In this chapter, we diverge from anecdotal report and move to theoretical foundation. To inform you about actions to improve parenting with an Aspie partner, I begin with Adam Smith's Empathy Imbalance Hypothesis of autism.

Empathy is a controversial subject in the field of AS/NT relationships. According to famed researcher Simon Baron-Cohen, those on the autism spectrum lack a theory of mind, or the ability to know what another person is thinking or feeling while at the same time knowing what you are thinking or feeling. If you are an NT, you have a theory of mind that guides you to empathize with others—even if you disagree with them—because you can see both sides of an issue. If you are an Aspie, this system is faulty. It is tough for Aspies to ascertain the minds of others and to empathize. Aspies frequently struggle to understand their own inner workings. Smith's research takes the theory of mind a step further. Through his Empathy Imbalance Hypothesis of autism, we come to understand why so many Aspies seem deeply moved by life experiences and yet are unable to relate well to others.

Some NTs say their Aspies are known for being socially clueless and even ruthless. Other NTs are adamant that their Aspie loved ones have deep, profoundly sensitive spirits and can relate emotionally to important issues.

Helen, an NT, her AS partner, Grant, and their twins, Jasmine and Jason, again take us into their daily lives. This time they help us find a very different way to look at empathy. *True empathy* is an integration of feelings and thoughts. What if *true empathy* is more multidimensional than empathizing with feelings (emotional empathy) or empathizing with facts (cognitive empathy)? And what if *true empathy* requires the ability to talk about this integration?

Can you soothe a child if they don't know you care?

Helen begins our session with a story. I've come to know that when Helen starts a session this way, she is coming from an unconscious place deep inside. She has an intuition, and she follows her hunch, recounting something seemingly unrelated. Out of these stories comes perspective that helps her to heal on her AS/NT parenting journey. We both learn from Helen's willingness to reveal the inner workings of her mind and heart.

Helen begins with a wistful look into the past.

As I drove past our old neighborhood the other day, I remembered a day I'd picked up Jasmine and Jason from school many years before. The twins had been about 7 then. At the spur of the moment I'd decided to take a detour through the new housing development going in next door

to our house. I'd thought the kids would enjoy seeing the earth-moving equipment, or watching the workers pour a foundation for a house. You know, it is kind of exciting to see a stretch of undeveloped land turn into houses, then a neighborhood.

I'd assumed Jason would enjoy the excursion, but I'd thought it would be particularly fun for Jasmine. You see Jasmine had a beloved children's story by P.D. Eastman, entitled, 'Are You My Mother?' Do you know the story? It's about a baby bird that falls from its nest and has to find its way home. You know how little ones love to read a story over and over again? Well Jasmine's favorite part was when the big red steam shovel gives a snort and carries the baby bird up to its nest at the top of the tree and back to its mother. From the first time she read that book—and she taught herself to read before kindergarten you know—well from the very first time she read it, she would point to backhoes and Bobcats and call them 'snorts.' It was so cute. She used to invent all kinds of words for things. Snort is what we called any earth-moving machine . . . . So you see, I'd been very sure she would enjoy seeing the snorts working on the housing project. As we'd turned into the project, I'd been pleased that I could share this little moment with my children. I'd been happily anticipating Jasmine's delight at seeing snorts up close. But you will never guess what she said Dr. Marshack.

Helen looks at me with a Mona Lisa smile as she fondly remembered Jasmine as a little girl. The smile faded when she went on.

I was watching both children in the rearview mirror, expecting to see them both get all excited and giggle and point at the snorts. I was stunned to see that Jasmine looked alarmed. Her eyes widened and filled with tears. 'Mommy! Mommy!' she said anxiously. 'Why is the snort

raping Mother Nature?' Never mind her use of such a big word as 'rape.' She does things like that. But when she said that word, I noticed that there was a huge fir tree on the ground. I watched as the backhoe gouged huge mouthfuls of dirt from the side of a hill, scooping up the plants and rocks. Jasmine was seeing the scene a whole different way than I had anticipated. I was heartsick for her. I felt like a horrible mother for torturing her this way.

I pulled the car off the road and parked, so that I could turn around and comfort her. Jason was just fine about the snort. He thought the whole scene was 'really cool.' But Jasmine had sensed the violence of it all. A tree was wrenched alive from the earth and dropped unceremoniously to die. The snort destroyed the earth home of millions of little bugs and worms and rodents. How many birds' nests fell from that tree, leaving baby birds homeless, just like in the Eastman book? Jasmine was in such pain, and I couldn't help her. I offered a weak excuse that we have to move plants and earth to make space for houses for families to live in, but she was not convinced. The suffering was too great for her. I hugged her and offered that we would get out of this awful place as fast I could take us home, which calmed her only a little bit. I heard her muffled sobs all the way home.

Driving home, I looked nervously in my rearview mirror to be sure both kids were okay. Jason reached over from his big-kid car seat and lightly touched Jasmine's face with two fingers and said, 'It's okay Jazzie.' I almost lost it then myself. Jason has always been that way . . . a sweet little guy.

There are tears in Helen's eyes and a bit of pride in her voice as she ended her anecdote with Jason's empathic response to his sister.

Parenting Jasmine has been the most meaningful, frustrating, sad and disorienting experience of my life. On top of that, I have to deal with Grant, who is also an Aspie. I don't think anyone truly understands the chaos that reigns in our house. How am I to be there for Jasmine, comfort her from her daily anxieties, run interference for her with teachers, neighbors and friends and reinterpret for her the strange world she lives in, while at the same time doing it all for Grant? Good grief! Grant is supposed to help me, but he can only do that when everything is happy and calm. The least bit of distress, and he is 'gone,' one way or the other, just like Jasmine.

Can you imagine what he did when I told him of Jasmine's heartache over the tree? He gave me that usual vacant stare. Then slowly he offered this sage advice, 'Oh she'll get over it.' Dr. Marshack, the reason I am telling you this is that it is no different today with Grant or Jasmine than it was all those years ago with the snorts. Grant and I are so disconnected emotionally. Now I realize that it is happening with Jasmine, too . . . and I am afraid of losing her. How on earth can I soothe Jasmine and offer parenting support at difficult times like this. . . and help her grow to independence when she and Grant don't recognize that I care about them or have my own feelings, too?

Helen has that same look I have seen so often when she tells me these stories, a combination of fatigue, heartache, loneliness and fear.

Emotions without empathy are just FEELINGS

Helen is a strong and compassionate woman. She really does understand the sufferings and joys of her daughter and husband. She understands her NT son, Jason, too. She has this extraordinary capacity to empathize with most people even when it is very painful to do so. This is probably why she is a successful naturopathic physician. It's one thing to know your science, to be able to diagnose and prescribe appropriate treatments. It's quite another to fully engage in the healing process through a powerful empathic connection with patients. Researchers tell us that a huge part of the healing process is believing in yourself and your healer. Because Helen possesses both medical training and this kind of deep empathy, she has a huge following of happy, healthy patients. She's a remarkable healer.

Helen knows she is an exceptional healer, yet she struggles to heal her own child. Helen knows that she can read people very well. She knows that she is brave and can help patients who are in pain without fatiguing herself by taking on too much worry for them. She has the ability to understand herself at the same time that she understands the other person. She can transition back and forth without thinking about it. This ability is well defined by Simon Baron-Cohen as theory of mind.[18] Despite her healing skills, Helen cannot reach her daughter. She had not been able to readily ease Jasmine's pain over the violent upheaval she witnessed that day in the housing development. No amount of love or empathy ever seems to reach Jasmine. Once Jasmine is reverberating with feelings, she cannot be reasoned with. The pain runs its course until Jasmine tires out, or worse—spirals into depression or a meltdown.

"You know Helen," I say, "There might be another way to look at this situation that could bring you some comfort. The other day I was reading an interesting journal article by Adam Smith, a researcher from Scotland.[19] He has a theory that may help explain these conundrums

---

18   Baron-Cohen, Simon. "Understanding other minds: Perspectives from developmental cognitive neuroscience." In *Theory of mind and autism: A fifteen year review*, edited by S. Baron-Cohen, H. Tager-Flusberg & D.J. Cohen, 2000, (3-20). Oxford England: Oxford University Press.

19   Smith, Adam. "The Empathy Imbalance Hypothesis of Autism: A Theoretical Approach to Cognitive and Emotional Empathy in Autistic Development," *The Psychological Record, 2009, (59) 273-294.*

you find yourself in with Jasmine and Grant. I know you don't want to hear just another not-very-helpful theory of Asperger's, but this theory leads to some practical ideas that might work with your family. It kind of explains why all of your love and empathy don't seem to reach Jasmine when she is really distraught, such as the time you took her to see the snorts. Because Jasmine and Grant lack a theory of mind, they also lack *true empathy*. Without empathy, emotions are just FEELINGS . . . in capital letters. It is hard for Jasmine and Grant to hear your words and change their focus when their feelings are overwhelming them. Do you want to know more?" Helen nods her approval, ever hopeful there is a way into the unfathomable world of Jasmine's mind and heart—and back out again to sanity.

Theory of mind is only one half of empathy

The theory of mind postulates that people with Asperger Syndrome have some degree of mind blindness, or an inability to fathom the motivations and feelings of others. Aspies don't seem to read the social clues that tell NTs what is going on. For example, Aspies are notoriously poor at recognizing complex emotions in others. They struggle to understand that someone may be stretching the truth for emphasis or as the punch line to a joke. They are confused by irony, pretense, metaphor, deception, faux pas, white lies and so forth. This is why NTs find Aspies to be clueless in social situations and why there are all types of curricula on the subject of teaching Aspies how to navigate the social world.

Smith's research takes this theory of mind a step further. I think it explains Jasmine's extreme distress at watching the violent destruction of the earth. The Empathy Imbalance

> . . .many Aspies seem deeply moved by life experiences and yet are unable to relate to others . . . .because they cannot get out of one kind of empathy and into the other.

Hypothesis of autism explains why so many Aspies seem deeply moved by life experiences and yet are unable to relate well to others. It's not really that Jasmine and Grant aren't able to empathize. Rather it is because they cannot easily move between the two kinds of empathy, even if a loving person tries to help them do so.

What are these two kinds of empathy? According to Smith, the first type is emotional empathy (EE) and is exemplified by Jasmine's heart-wrenching pain at witnessing the raping of the land by the unfeeling snort. In her mind, the snort was mercilessly killing the tree and destroying the homes of many animals, including baby birds. EE is just that: It's feeling without thought. It is the punch to the gut that we feel when we are horrified. It is also the exuberance that we feel when we witness an uncommonly beautiful sight, such as a full rainbow. It is the ability to feel the feelings of another whether or not we understand those feelings. The emotions are there. The tears flow. The blood rushes to our face. Our heart beats faster. It is an experience that fills the entire moment to the brim of our being. For Aspies this moment spills over into everything and onto everyone around them.

The other type of empathy is cognitive empathy (CE). It is exemplified by Helen's response to Jasmine. Helen didn't expect her daughter to be distressed by watching the snorts. She anticipated that her daughter would delight in the detour to the housing development. When it didn't work out that way, Helen quickly shifted her attention to Jasmine's suffering. She was able to recognize her daughter's emotional pain and see that, for Jasmine, it was a terrifying experience of violence. CE is the analytical side of empathy, or what Baron-Cohen means by theory of mind. Helen has good social radar, or theory of mind; hence she can instantly recognize her daughter's (and her son, Jason's,) emotional response to the construction scene.

But it doesn't stop there. Smith suggests that NTs have a good balance or interplay of CE and EE, whereas Aspies do not. Helen was able to recognize her daughter's distress and understand where it was coming from, which is CE. She also was able to feel Jasmine's feelings and to really know how awful her daughter felt, which is EE. By combining EE and CE, Helen was able to put her own needs aside for the moment and reach out to comfort her daughter. Helen was able to hold her own reality in one hand and Jasmine's in another while making a bridge between the two. That bridge was words, Helen's comforting words, supportive words, warm and loving words, words that let Jasmine know her mother knew what she was feeling and cared.

This imbalance in EE and CE is not just a difference between adult and child. Jason also was able to empathize with his sister. We can't be sure that he recognized what upset her, but at age 7 he was using EE and CE. He'd understood Jasmine was distressed, and he'd wanted to help her. Helen has other stories of how sweet and sensitive and well-liked Jason is, so I suspect his balance of empathy is well integrated. But what about Grant? He is an adult with Asperger Syndrome. When his wife had told him what had happened that afternoon, he had missed the point entirely. Or rather he'd missed several points.

Without CE, Grant was unable to understand what motivated Helen to tell him this story. He couldn't see that it was more than just a story about Jasmine and Jason and the snorts. It was even more than the story of Jasmine's pain. It was Helen's story, too. Helen was reeling from her own emotions. She needed to debrief a stressful parenting moment. She needed Grant's emotional support to reassure her that she was a good mommy. She also needed to brainstorm a bit about Jasmine's unusual reaction. Grant's response was one-sided and devoid of any empathy. Helen didn't even get to the part of the story about Jason's kindness toward his crying sister. Grant's perfunctory announcement that Jasmine would "get over it" stopped Helen in her tracks. How could she continue with her tender story when her husband saw it as inconsequential?

Helen takes her job as a parent very seriously. She believes that her job is to help both Jason and Jasmine discover who they are and grow into all that they can be. On the trip home from school that day, Helen learned something about her daughter that she hadn't known. She'd sensed it was important—this disconnect between feeling and thinking. Clearly Jasmine has deep emotional responses. But she has few ways to regulate or speak to those responses through her own mental reasoning. It's even difficult for Jasmine to accept her mother's soothing because she doesn't understand the intent of soothing.

The disconnect between cognitive empathy and emotional empathy defines Asperger Syndrome

Helen is wide eyed with excitement as she explains her thoughts.

Dr. Marshack this makes so much sense. But I think there is more. I get it that there are two types of empathy, cognitive and emotional. And I get that Jasmine and Grant struggle to get out of emotional empathy when they are over-stimulated, but I wonder if the problem is the transition. You know I wonder if they do have cognitive empathy, too. It's just that they are not connected up in their brains like we are.

"Tell me more Helen," I say. "I think you are onto something."
Helen continues.

Well it is just that Jasmine is much more than a bundle of uncontrolled feelings. She has deep and profound insight, too, so I know she can empathize. For example, when she was 11 she came to me with a question. Even then she listened to National Public Radio (NPR). Isn't that just so odd, but that is Jasmine for you. She never has had the same interests as other girls her age. I guess she likes gathering information. She was listening to a debate on the topic of legalizing euthanasia for terminally ill people. Even weirder right? So she asked me about it one evening. Her question was kind of vague. She said, 'Mom, what's this about euthanasia?'

I was taken aback at first. Even though I gave birth to this child and have lived with her many years, she never ceases to amaze me. I also know that answering a question like that requires a bit more of me. Plus I know there is more to Jasmine's question than first appears. I thought carefully for a moment and then I said, 'What do you think?'

Jasmine clearly understood what euthanasia is and summed it up nicely when she said, 'I can't imagine why there is all this debate about making it legal when a person should have the right to decide if they want to die. If they are so sick that keeping them alive is torture, then why would you have to vote on something like that?'

Jasmine didn't ask me for my opinion exactly, but she did want to talk about this phenomenon of taking a vote on human rights. Cleary this is an example of cognitive empathy, don't you think?

"I have to agree with you Helen," I say.
Helen is on a roll and takes my comment as permission to continue.

Now the interesting thing is that Jasmine can comprehend a complex social issue, such as legalizing euthanasia, but she doesn't discuss the emotional components of the issue. She is clear and focused on the merits of the issue, not how people may feel about it. She is somewhat empathetic to the person who is suffering and dying and may want to elect euthanasia, but only because she feels that is their right, like a Constitutional right or something. But she doesn't mention a word about how others may feel about this controversial subject. No thought about the religious views, or how the families may feel, or what a difficult spot this puts the physician in. It's like she has cognitive empathy, too, but without a connection to the emotional empathy. So she misses the bigger picture.

Helen has another look of inspiration.

Gosh this is exactly what Grant did to me that day of the snort. He got it that Jasmine would 'get over it,' but he missed the emotional implications. So I think what goes on is that Aspies can experience cognitive empathy when they are calm, cool and collected. And they can experience emotional empathy when they are aroused by something startling or important to them. I don't think they put the two together very well. Don't you think there is the important step of integrating cognitive and emotional empathy in order to understand and relate to the total experience?

It is so like Helen to figure this out. This is a woman who is comfortable with both types of empathy and easily navigates the social world to provide healing and nurturing on a daily basis. Plus who better to explain Smith's hypothesis than a woman who is a mom to an Aspie and a wife to an Aspie. Psychologists should definitely listen more to moms. I tell her, "Helen, I shouldn't be amazed at your discovery since you are a poster child for empathy. You have taken this theory right into the practical world for those of you who live with Aspies."

Alexithymia short-circuits empathy

Helen is connecting the dots like crazy.

A couple of years after the euthanasia discussion, Grant and I had to tell the children that Grant's mother was very ill and dying. She had a long-term illness, so we knew this would happen sooner or later. Grandma and Grandpa lived in another state, and we saw them only once a year, but we did have the usual phone calls. The twins loved their grandparents, but they weren't close, because they hadn't grown up with them [nearby] like they have my family.

Grandma had been in and out of the hospital several times and had had a couple of major surgeries. They were horrendous surgeries, too. She'd had to have one leg amputated. A year later the other leg had been amputated. It was awful. I couldn't believe she'd survived the first amputation, so I was absolutely certain she wouldn't make it through the second one. With each surgery, I'd told Grant that he should make more time with his mother. I'd suggested that he should take an emergency leave of absence from work and fly out to see her. Do you know what he said, Dr. Marshack? Oh my goodness. He said, 'Well I am sure Mom or Dad will call if it is that urgent.' No kidding. The woman has her leg cut off to save her life, and Grant can't see it is urgent. No empathy of either kind was in operation as far as I can tell. I guess because he wasn't having his leg amputated, he didn't feel the emotional or physical pain. Or perhaps he couldn't imagine that it was serious, because no one had officially told him so. I'd told him, but he thinks I overreact to everything.

As it turned out, shortly after this second amputation, Grant's mother got a terrible infection that raged through her body. That started shutting down one body organ after another. She must have been in terrible pain and very frightened. She had always been a vivacious redhead, who loved parties and people. Once again I'd urged Grant to take an emergency leave of absence and fly out that very night to visit his mother. I'd told him that I could make arrangements for the children's care and fly there the next day to help him. Once again he made the same bizarre statement, 'I'm sure Dad will call if it is urgent.'

I couldn't believe my ears. I'd said, 'Grant. I don't think you understand. Your mother is dying. She has had two horrible, desperate life-saving surgeries this past year, and she is not going to make it this time. I am a doctor. Please believe me. Her body is shutting down. They won't be able to stop the infection. Her body can't handle the damage and recover any longer. You simply must go home to see her one last time.' I was desperate for Grant. I know this man. I know he doesn't understand these emotional things or gets stuck or something. I worried that he would feel horrible later if he didn't go to his mother and his father now. Both of them needed him. But he'd refused.

In a few days Grandma was in a coma and on life support. We didn't tell the children everything over this period of time, but we did tell them that Grandma was very ill and might die. I didn't want them to be surprised or to feel betrayed, because we hadn't kept them informed. But I couldn't bear to tell them about her amputations. It was too gruesome, and I didn't want them to have nightmares.

Eventually we got the call from Grandpa. He'd been very upset of course. I remember telling Grant that we had to tell the children everything now. We sat down at the table, and I waited for Grant to start. He was speechless. I held his hand and looked at him again, hoping to make eye contact and to encourage him to take the lead. He wouldn't look at me or the twins. I gathered my courage and took over. I said, 'Jasmine . . . Jason . . .you both know that Grandma has been very ill and in the hospital.' They both just looked at me with non-blinking eyes. 'I have something sad to tell you.' The kids didn't move a muscle. 'We just heard from Grandpa. The doctors have advised him to take Grandma off life support. She is dying and suffering. She is unconscious and not able to make her own choices anymore. The doctors told Grandpa that she will not regain consciousness and will die a painful death if they don't help her.'

I looked at Grant and squeezed his hand, giving him a loving signal that I was there to help him if he wanted to take over the conversation. Again he did nothing. Jason was on the edge of his chair, waiting for me to finish. He knew somehow that there was more. I couldn't read Jasmine, though. She looked thoughtful, like she was weighing every word carefully. I continued, 'What this means is that the doctors will give Grandma morphine ,so she can go into a deep sleep and not feel the pain of death. They will take her off all of her IVs, her medicine and food . . . and the machine that helps her breathe and keeps her heart beating. Then she will die very shortly, because her body cannot take care of her anymore.'

It seemed like it took hours to have this short, one-sided conversation. It was only a few minutes of time really. I remember I felt as though I was holding my breath. I was doing that again just now as I told the story. It was one of the most difficult times in my life. When I finished I took a deep breath and I waited. No one said a thing. It was as if the whole family was spellbound and waiting for something or someone. Me? I think so. At important times like this they all wait for me to tell them what to do. I squeezed Grant's hand again, realizing that he was so overwhelmed he could not function very well. They all needed me to help them know what to do or say next. I said, 'Jason, Jasmine, I know you must be having some strong feelings right now. Do you want to tell Dad and me what you are feeling and thinking about Grandma?'

Once permission was given to express himself, Jason burst into tears and screamed, 'No! No! I don't want Grandma to die. No! No! Can't they keep her on life support a little longer? Maybe she will pull through.' Then he looked at me from across the table with those beautiful eyes full of tears, imploring me for comfort. I reached my hand across the table toward Jason, still holding Grant's hand with my other. Jason's fingers reached out to touch mine. Our eyes met, and we both wept for a moment.

My heart was breaking for Jason. I said, 'I know honey. I know.' I didn't have to explain more to Jason. He understood that there was no way to save Grandma. At that moment he let go of her, safe in the knowledge that he was not alone, and that I would help him grieve.

When Jasmine heard her brother's outburst and saw my empathic response to him, she looked puzzled. Now that I better understand cognitive and emotional empathy, I realize why Jasmine said what she said next. Jasmine was locked into a mental state, not an emotional one. She wasn't all that concerned about her grandmother. It was similar to how her father had reacted when he first learned of Grandmother's surgeries. Leg amputations were foreign to him, unheard of. Jasmine seemed unmoved by her brother's crying or by the fact that I had a huge lump in my throat. She seemed oblivious of Grant, who was so overpowered by his own feelings of loss that he sat there lifeless. Given all of this, is it any surprise that Jasmine said, 'Why do you want the doctors to keep Grandma on life support and make her suffer more?' Don't you see Dr. Marshack?

Helen looks at me intently, waiting for an expression that indicates I "got it," that I really "got it!" She can see the excited interest on my face, so she continues. "You got it," she says and smiles confidently.

Jasmine already knew about euthanasia from NPR. She could handle this transition better than she'd handled the snort and the tree—even though her Grandmother's death had to be far more distressing for her. It wasn't new. It wasn't startling. She'd known Grandma was sick and might die. She just hadn't known when. When we finally told Jasmine, she accepted it with cognitive empathy. But she could not transition back to EE and be empathic for her brother or her dad or me—or even for herself.

I didn't explain it to Helen then, but her story is a perfect, albeit a sad, example of alexithymia, or the inability of Aspies to talk about their feelings. Just as there is a disconnect between cognitive and emotional empathy, Aspies have a disconnect between what they are feeling and the words to describe their feelings. This is especially so when the situation is grim, such as the pending death of Grant's mother.

Undoubtedly Grant was shocked at the news that his mother would die. Still, he was unable to express his feelings with words in spite of Helen's support and invitations to talk. Jasmine could sum things up nicely in a detached way, because she was not registering emotional empathy for her grandmother, her father, her mother, her brother or herself. However, in one short emotional outburst, Jason had spoken to all of them. His distress over his grandmother's death was not just about his loss but about the loss to all of them. As Helen has discovered, *true empathy* is a complex and dynamic interplay of emotional empathy, cognitive empathy and words.

The whole is more than the sum of the parts, but you still have to break it down for Aspies

In a moment of insight, Helen had explained a complex theory from the perspective of one who lives it. She lives daily with a partner and a child who have Asperger Syndrome; hence she knows firsthand how it feels to be an NT caught in the Aspie no-man's-land—that place between cognitive empathy and emotional empathy. This is the kind of anecdotal information that often escapes researchers.

Smith eloquently describes the two major types of empathy, and he notes that a person can have varying degrees of each. Only someone such as Helen could see that there is an entirely different dimension when cognitive and emotional empathy don't interact. For example, if Grant or Jasmine cannot integrate CE and EE in one encounter, then their experience of empathy is flat. Is it really empathy if you only have feelings, or you only have thoughts? Is it really empathy if you cannot talk about your feelings or those of another? In other words, is the problem an imbalance in the two types of empathy, or is the problem the missing link that integrates the two types—that link that allows a smooth transition between CE and EE?

Smith's theory can help us better understand the behaviors of Aspies caught in an emotional encounter that triggers empathy. With this understanding we may be able to devise methods to communicate across the AS/NT divide. Jasmine and Grant are both capable of cognitive empathy and emotional empathy, but not usually at the same time. They have devised a variety of coping mechanisms to deal with this disconnect.

We know that transitions are difficult for those on the autism spectrum. When Jasmine saw the tree torn from the ground and the earth gouged from the hillside, she had to make an abrupt transition from a fun outing to a violent and unexpected scene. As a result her EE overwhelmed her, and she could do no more than cry. Her brother, on the other hand, could make the transition from a fun outing to demonstrating EE and CE for his sister. Jasmine does not have the skills to move from her over-aroused emotional state to a more detached intellectual understanding of the situation. If she could make that leap, she would be better able to cope with lots of emotional transitions.

Grant was so overly aroused by the prospect of his mother's death that he totally cut himself off from his feelings. Nor was he able to speak about them. Smith suggests that those on the autism spectrum actually feel their emotions more intensely than the rest of us. Perhaps. Or could it be that without the quick regulation of EE by CE, their feelings have nowhere to go except to reverberate and become even more intense? To protect themselves from this intensity, Aspies shut down completely. Grant may have been so upset about his mother's death that he couldn't talk or look into his wife's eyes. He couldn't comfort his children either. Many, many people with AS avoid eye contact even in normal daily encounters. They report the intense emotion that comes from eye contact is painful, so they avoid it. This leaves the NTs in their lives believing the Aspie doesn't care or isn't listening.

It is natural for NTs with high EE and CE to reach out to others to get or give comfort. Sharing one's feelings or asking about the other person's feelings is part of relating for NTs. Not so for Aspies. Grant could not talk about his mother. He wouldn't listen to his wife try to coach him about his mother's pending death. He was so overwhelmed emotionally that he could not reach across the divide to use his cognitive empathy. He couldn't see that his wife needed to talk with him. He couldn't see that his children needed him. He couldn't see that his mother and father needed him either. Not everyone goes home one last time to be with a dying parent, but Grant could not even explain why he wasn't going. The best reason he could come up with was that his parents hadn't told him it was time to go home yet. Whether Grant could not connect the dots and understand that his mother was dying and that his family needed him (CE), or he could not express his feelings (EE), he was not able to communicate with his family . . . and get or give support.

What is clearly missing for both Grant and Jasmine is a link between cognitive and emotional empathy. The type of empathy with which they first respond will determine their reaction. Cold and analytical responses emerge when Jasmine discusses euthanasia without the benefit and warmth of emotional empathy. Self absorption into a non-verbal state emerges when Grant learns that his mother's death is imminent. He has no way to use the rationale of cognitive empathy to balance his overwhelming emotional empathy.

Helen, and to some extent Jason, acts as the connecting link between the two empathies for Grant and Jasmine. It is a confusing burden for mother and son. The theories discussed in this and the next two chapters should make their job a bit easier. The major problem for Aspies who get stuck in their feelings or stuck in their thoughts is that they have no guidance about doing anything else. Had Helen known about EE and CE, she could have prepared Jasmine for the trip to see the snorts. What if she had told Jasmine that they would be able to see a real snort at work, digging into the ground and clearing the land of trees so that a new house could be built? Considering how much Jasmine adored this children's book, Helen could have surmised that Jasmine would have lots of EE around the story, particularly for the little bird and the snort. Perhaps Helen could have emphasized that real life isn't like a children's story and that real snorts don't actually rescue lost baby birds. Jasmine would have been better prepared for the scene. She may still have felt empathy for the dying tree, but she and her mother could have talked about the contrast between the storybook and reality.

A very similar solution could have worked for Helen and Grant. Helen and Grant might have sought psychotherapy together prior to his mother's death. A psychologist could have helped Grant reason through what was happening to him and to his mother. An objective professional could have put words to the emotions that were welling up inside of Grant. With practice in therapy, he and Helen may have been able to talk about the events to come and planned a course of action. The sudden emotional transition Grant faced with the death of his mother could have been avoided.

It may seem unfair that Helen must be, for Grant and Jasmine, the bridge between the worlds of emotional empathy and cognitive empathy. Certainly working with a psychologist(s) helps. If you have committed to a life with an Aspie partner, if you love him or her and want it all to work out, being the bridge is your assignment. I also think that you will have a very grateful Aspie when he or she finally comprehends the extra work you do to smooth these tough transitions. With therapy this awareness is possible.

Lessons learned

1. There is more to empathy than meets the eye. It is a complex system of emotional empathy and cognitive empathy and multiple transitions between the two.

2. Most NTs make the transition between emotional empathy and cognitive empathy very easily, thus striking a balance between the two. This is difficult for Aspies to accomplish. Mainly because they lack a theory of mind, or the ability to empathize even when disagreeing.

3. Aspies get stuck in one form of empathy or another and need help making the transition to a more productive emotional outcome. NTs' mastery of CE, EE and words enables them to help Aspies create *true empathy*.

4. NT family members will be relied on to help their Aspie loved ones make these transitions. Don't be too hard on yourself if you cannot anticipate every possible roadblock for the Aspie.

5. Aspies need to appreciate their NT partners for the exceptional work the NTs do to keep the communication going.

6. Always have a good psychologist in your hip pocket. One way to reduce the emotional overload for Aspies and NTs alike is to have a calming and knowledgeable professional(s) to help you sort things out.

CHAPTER FIVE

Out of Brain – Out of Mind

Helen and NTs like her are coming to understand how their Asperger Syndrome loved ones think. Helen notices patterns and discusses her insights with her psychologist. She is also developing adaptations to the Aspie world: Some are healthy, others less so. But adaptation is not enough for Helen and the others you'll meet in this chapter. They want to know WHY their Aspies act this way. Neuro-typicals (NTs) repeatedly ask, "Why can't she SEE what I am saying?" Or they ask, "Why can't he CONNECT with my feelings?" It is not hard to see the pattern in these "Why?" questions. NTs repeatedly seek a mutually satisfying solution, not the one-sided, systemic model acceptable to their Aspies.

Helen got some answers to her questions when she learned about Adam Smith's Empathy Imbalance Hypothesis, described in the preceding chapter.[20] She quickly recognized that her Aspies have a huge disconnect between thinking and feeling, or cognitive empathy (CE) and emotional empathy (EE). But what is the cause of this disconnect? That's the real WHY question. According to the latest neuroscience research discussed in Simon Baron-Cohen's exciting new book, *The Science of Evil: On Empathy and the Origins of Evil*,[21] the cause is poorly working empathy circuits in the brain. The Aspie brain has limited neurological mechanisms in place to understand or empathize with the NT. We've been emphasizing that Aspies cannot "see" what is not in their mind. Another way to understand the Aspie's lack of empathy from a neurological perspective is "out of brain- out of mind."

In this second of the three chapters on theory, you will learn why no matter how much we explain or teach or train the Aspie mind, certain neurological circuits don't work as they do in the NT brain. Baron-Cohen shows us there is more to empathy than CE and EE. He points to a huge array of empathy circuits designed to interconnect to create a complex spectrum of empathy.

Empathy disorders

Baron-Cohen offers a new way to look at Asperger Syndrome. Through the lens of recent neuroscience and DNA research, he postulates that some psychiatric disorders result from faulty empathy circuits in the brain. Multiple empathy circuits contribute to cognitive empathy and emotional empathy; hence Baron-Cohen proposes that we categorize Asperger's diagnoses as empathy disorders. (I won't go into all of the brain research—and wouldn't even if I could tell the difference

20   Smith, Adam. "The Empathy Imbalance Hypothesis of Autism: A Theoretical Approach to Cognitive and Emotional Empathy in Autistic Development," *Psychological Record* (2009), 273-294.

21   Baron-Cohen, Simon. (2011). *The Science of Evil: On Empathy and the Origins of Evil*. New York: Basic Books, Inc.

between the dorsal medial prefrontal cortex, the frontal operculum and the amygdala. There is a way to understand this stuff even if you are not a brain surgeon, but I'll get to that later.)

First, let's meet some couples who are AS/NT co-parents, and who exemplify the problem inherent to empathy disorders and parenting.

As usual, Adrienne and Stefan arrive early for their appointment, but Adrienne looks grim.

"You look distressed Adrienne," I say. "Is there something on your mind?"

"Oh yes, but why not let Stefan tell you? I can't believe he could be so cruel!" Adrienne glares at Stefan.

Calmly, Stefan takes up the verbal prompt and begins to explain. "Well Dr. Marshack, Adrienne is upset with me, because I wouldn't help her take the cat to the vet. I tried to explain that I have a very heavy day at work, and I just can't call in sick for a cat."

Before I can respond, Adrienne jumps in. "Oh that's not it, and you know it! All I asked of you is **if** you could go **with** me to the vet, because I was upset about Mr. Puddin'. He has been in our family for 15 years, and we are all very attached to him. I know he is getting older, and I worry. When I saw him losing weight, not eating and acting kind of sick, I got scared. I knew I needed to take him to the vet, but I was afraid of what she would tell me. Plus I worry that the kids will freak out if they think their 'baby' is going to die. But noooooo. All you could think of was work—as usual. Work is far more important than your family." Adrienne sits there tight-lipped and smug with righteous anger.

Stefan interrupts his wife with an explanation, "Yes, but I told you that I couldn't get away from work and that wasn't good enough for you. I told you to take the cat to the vet. I didn't try to stop you."

"Ohhhhhhhhhh," exclaims Adrienne, "You make me so crazy when you say things like that. Why don't you tell Dr. Marshack what you actually said Stefan?"

Again very calmly, as if pulling out a list of items for the grocery story, Stefan offers the facts. "Oh I know what you mean. I said, 'He's only a cat.'"

"Oh my God! Yes!" Adrienne exclaims. "You said, 'He's only a cat' as if your work is more important than me and the kids. What am I supposed to tell them . . . that their Daddy is a cruel man who could care less about their pet's suffering?"

At that point both fall silent. Stefan stares off blankly and shifts in his seat, waiting for his next verbal prompt. Adrienne looks at me imploringly. Clearly she needs some affirmation that her husband is a heartless dolt. But I try another tack. "Adrienne, Stefan: Let me help you. There might be another way to look at this. First of all, tell me Adrienne, is your cat okay?"

"Yes, Dr. Marshack. Thank you for asking." Adrienne launches into a long explanation of Mr. Puddin's maladies. She is so relieved to have an empathic listener that she pours out her heart. "He has to take medicine now for the rest of his life, but I don't mind, and the children are so relieved!" I let her explain for a minute or two, then gently nudge her to let it be for awhile.

Rather than confuse Stefan even more with the convoluted logic of his NT wife, I start by asking him a few questions, and I verbally guide him in the empathy process. "Stefan, are you aware that your wife is fond of Mr. Puddin' and that she even feels like he was her first 'baby'?" Stefan nods affirmatively.

"And can you imagine that Adrienne was just heartsick when she saw her 'baby' getting sicker and sicker?" Again Stefan agrees.

"Furthermore," I continue, "I bet she was also afraid to take the cat to the vet, because she kind of wanted to avoid the potential bad news." Stefan waivers and stiffens, showing some disapproval with my interpretation, so I clarify. "What I mean by this is that sometimes we just kind of freeze emotionally when we have to do something we really don't want to do." Stefan relaxes and accepts my explanation.

"Now here's what I think happened. I don't really think that Adrienne meant for you to take off from work to help her take the cat to the vet, although she might have liked that," I say. "What she was really asking for was emotional support. She just wanted you to let her know you cared and realized how important this was to her. Maybe you could have said, 'Honey if I could get away from work I would. I know you are worried sick about Mr. Puddin'. He's been in our family for years. Be brave. I am sure the vet will have answers for you. As soon as you know anything please call me on my cell. Okay? Love you Honey.' "

Stefan's face brightens as he feels that I understand and support him. He responds, "Yes, that's what I meant!"

Adrienne snarls back. "Like hell you did! You said, 'It's only a cat!' Then you just drove off to work. How could you?" Stefan's look of optimism fades.

I step in again. "Adrienne, if you let me finish, I think this will finally make some sense." Adrienne concedes reluctantly.

"So I want to ask you a question Stefan. When you said, 'It's only a cat,' did you mean that comment as a statement of support? I mean, did you think the cat's situation shouldn't be as distressing as the serious illness of a person, say Adrienne's sister or a close friend?"

Stefan looks at me with interest and a sense of relief at being understood. "Yes," he says. "I was just trying to help, but I guess I said the wrong thing."

Adrienne's look softens with the insight into her husband. I continue, "Adrienne, try to remember that you and Stefan have very different ways that you process information. You are a master at empathy, but Stefan is not. His empathy circuits are arranged differently, because he has Asperger's. He loves you. He knows you are upset. However, he doesn't recognize that your request for him to take time off from work is a metaphor for giving you emotional support. He does his best to support you by speaking to the facts. Fact number one, his employer will not let him take time off from work. Fact number two, you will recover from the loss of your cat, which of course you know is true."

"Yes Dr. Marshack," says Adrienne, "I realize this is true, but is that really the best he can do? I know this makes sense . . . that Stefan just wanted to help, and logic is his kind of help. But will he ever be able to speak to my feelings? Will he always be like this? How do I teach the children compassion when their father ignores their feelings?" Adrienne looks hopeless and starts to cry.

This is the conundrum isn't it? To an NT, empathy is key to love and connectedness and really "seeing" who the other person is. But this is precisely the area in which Aspies fail time and time again. Having the answer to why Stefan didn't make an empathic response helps Adrienne recognize that her husband cares. Still, it is not the same as *true empathy* in the moment when it is needed.

Read the dialogue again. Notice that Stefan could not speak unless instructed to do so when I asked him a specific question. Notice that I had to act as a guide for Stefan through the empathy process. I guided Stefan to "light up" his separate empathy circuits much like a pilot or flight attendant turns on floor lights that lead to emergency exits in airplanes. Once the lights were turned on, and the circuits were connected, Stefan understood his wife—and himself— better. He could actually offer an empathic response. He said, "I was just trying to help, but I guess I said the wrong thing."

To answer Adrienne's question, "Will he always be like this?" Maybe. Researchers and clinicians aren't sure. There are some promising therapies. So far we really have as little information on successful clinical interventions as we do on the genetic and neurological structure of the brain. For now the bottom line is that Adrienne and other NTs need to turn on the lights for their Aspie mates and children. Helping Aspies through the mysterious world of non-verbal and verbal empathy is not so stressful if NTs don't take it personally. It is equally true that Aspie co-parents must accept coaching by their NT spouse as well as by the family psychologist. That requires a great deal of love and acceptance on the Aspie's part.

True empathy is like a dimmer switch

Think Chevy Chase and the movie "Christmas Vacation." Chase's character, Clark Griswold, strung hundreds of Christmas lights on his house to welcome the holidays. He checked every bulb on each string of lights before stapling them to his roof. When he plugged the house extension cord into the last in a long string of Christmas light cords, nothing happened. When his wife Ellen (played by Barbara De'Angelo) figured out that there was a master switch in the garage, she flipped it, and power surged to the Christmas lights.

We've probably all experienced the frustration of hanging Christmas lights (In our house we call them Chanukah lights.), only to find that one string doesn't work. Is there a bulb burned out? Are all the bulbs screwed in properly? Does a string need a fuse? Is the wiring damaged? If we can't successfully problem solve, we might give up, buy more strings of lights and start over. But we can't do that with our brains. The brain has a number of circuits that are all connected up like Christmas lights. If one part doesn't work right, then the rest of the circuits malfunction, too. Plus these brain circuits are so tightly integrated that multiple circuits depend upon multiple other circuits to carry out sophisticated human behaviors and to comprehend complex thoughts and feelings. Our brains are truly amazing.

Some of these brain circuits are specifically wired for empathy.

> The brain has a number of circuits that are all connected up like Christmas lights. If one part doesn't work right, then the rest of the circuits malfunction, too.

Many of these empathy circuits have been brain-mapped by neuroscientists, and they are discovering more circuits all the time.[22] Each circuit has its own particular empathic function and interacts with other circuits and other parts of the brain to produce a spectrum of empathy. Unlike Clark Griswold's Christmas lights, there is more than one switch that needs to turn on for empathy circuits to work. Many empathy circuits need to "light up" at the same time for the entire sequence of empathic communication to take place. For example, *true empathy* is the ability to be aware of one's own feelings and thoughts at the same time you are aware of another person's feelings and thoughts (or several other persons'). It means having the wherewithal to speak about this awareness. It also means creating mutual understanding and a sense of caring for one another. Wow! That is a lot of brain circuits to connect!

Let's get beyond the Christmas lights metaphor and look at a sampling of brain parts in the empathy circuits to learn what they actually do for us. Realize that each part is not so functional by itself, but needs the other circuits to carry out the complex empathy task of really stepping into the shoes of another person. For example, the medial prefrontal cortex (MPFC) compares your perspective to another person's perspective. The dorsal medial prefrontal cortex (dMPFC) helps us understand our own thoughts and feelings. The ventral medial prefrontal cortex (vMPFC) stores information about how strongly we feel about a course of action. The inferior frontal gyrus (IFG) helps with emotion recognition.

Hang in there with me. There is no quiz at the end of the chapter. You don't have to memorize the parts of the brain. But I want you to have a sense of the complexity of these empathy circuits. To continue then, the caudal anterior cingulate cortex (CACC) is activated with pain: Not just when you feel pain but when you observe pain in others.

---

22   Brain mapping has most recently been in the news as President Obama committed federal dollars to map the brain so that we can find better treatments for a variety of health disorders such as Alzheimers and autism.

The anterior insula (AI) is involved in bodily self awareness, something that is tied to empathy. The right temporoparietal junction (RTPJ) helps us judge another person's intentions and beliefs.

I discussed the mirror neuron system in my book, *Going Over the Edge?*[23] This is the system of neurons that responds when we engage in an action and when we observe others engage in an action. For example, these neurons fire when we gaze in a certain direction or observe another person gaze in the same direction. Several parts of the brain, such as IFG and the inferior parietal lobule (IPL), are connected by the mirror neuron system. The interplay of these multiple and interacting empathy circuits is complicated. Your mirror neurons make you look in the same direction as the speaker, but you also need other empathy circuits to make meaning of why you are looking.

Most of you have heard of the amygdala, but you may not know that it is beneath the brain cortex in the limbic system. In a sense, it is a more primitive part of the brain. It plays a central role in empathy, because of its connection to fear. The amygdala cues us to look at someone's eyes to help us gather information about that person's emotions and intentions. People with Asperger Syndrome seem to avoid eye contact—unless they are specifically instructed, "Look me in the eye." Think of all the information that is lost by not looking into someone's eyes.

I have only named a few regions of the brain's empathy circuits to whet your appetite to learn more. All right, maybe not learn too much more. But are you getting the idea that our human brains are marvelously constructed? And pardon me if I erred in some way with my simplified descriptions of the brain. The point is that the empathy circuits in our brains are very complex. If a single one of them doesn't work, the whole network suffers—and so do our relationships.

---

23 Marshack, Kathy. (2009). *Going Over the Edge?* Kansas: Autism Asperger Publishing Co.

Your mirror neurons may signal you to mirror a speaker and look in the same direction he or she is looking (hence, "mirroring"). But these mirror neurons don't tell you why to look in the same direction. Your CACC may signal that another person is experiencing pain, but it doesn't signal you to speak about it—or give you a clue as to what to say. Unlike the Griswold family's straightforward strands of Christmas lights, the brain's empathy circuits must work together in a complex system, sending signals back and forth, to create an integrated and highly sophisticated "lights on" response. Remember, it is not empathy unless you respond appropriately to the other person.

Baron-Cohen believes that empathy is on a dimmer switch. How bright empathy burns depends on: life circumstances at any one time; which empathy circuits "light up;" which empathy circuits are working well; and other intervening factors, such as fatigue, hunger, sexual arousal, anxiety, and even how much alcohol is consumed. We experience more or less empathy on a spectrum of empathy, depending on these variables.

We all have a place on the empathy spectrum. NTs are higher on this spectrum than their Aspie partners. Even so, an NT's empathy can vary, As the research shows, those with Asperger Syndrome have only a few empathy circuits that work. Which ones are working define a particular empathy disorder. More about this later.

Turn the lights on

Jeremy wanted help turning the lights on for Lorri-Jane, his Aspie wife. Lorri-Jane is a devoted mother. She insists on a healthy diet for the entire family. She is very punctual and organized. The household runs like clockwork—even the children, who know darned good and well they better be on time for the school bus in the morning. But the kinder, more nurturing side of mothering seems to elude Lorri-Jane.

One morning Jeremy had been helping the children get going. He hadn't wanted them to miss the school bus. As his wife bustled by getting herself ready for work, he'd asked her if she wanted a slice of toast for breakfast. She'd politely declined, so Jeremy had put one slice in the toaster for his son Matt. The other children had wanted cereal. Then he thought again and put in a slice for himself. When Lorri-Jane came through the kitchen again she'd exploded, "Why are you wasting toast when I told you I didn't want any?"

Jeremy was stunned. Lorri-Jane had seen the children sitting at the table, two with cereal bowls and Matt with an empty plate waiting for his eggs and toast. Yet she couldn't compute that Jeremy was helping the children with breakfast. Secondly, she couldn't compute that the toast was for anyone other than herself—and she didn't want any. Third, she accused Jeremy of "wasting" toast. To make matters worse, when Jeremy explained that he was making toast for Matt, and for himself, Lorri-Jane shrugged matter-of-factly and said, "Why didn't you tell me?" Then she walked away without an apology, leaving Jeremy and the children struggling with their emotional upset over what had just happened.

I have explained to Jeremy that there are probably a number of empathy circuits not working effectively in Lorri-Jane's brain. He knows that she loves the children, or she wouldn't work so hard to have everything they need. He knows that she loves him, too, because she is concerned about his health. But it feels like abuse to Jeremy when Lorri-Jane accuses him of wrongdoing and never apologizes for her missteps.

Can you see how important these multiple interacting empathy circuits are in daily life? Can you see how unpleasant life can get when the simplest of things is misunderstood? How does Jeremy explain to his son that Mommy didn't realize he wanted toast? I guess Matt could accept that Mommy didn't know he was having toast, but how does he make sense of her abusive retort? Do you really think that a little boy will accept the explanation that Mommy's mirror neuron system slipped—or that her RTPJ wasn't working that morning? Of course not. Matt takes it personally, probably believing that he should forgo toast from now on, so that Mommy doesn't get mad.

So how does Jeremy help his wife turn up the dimmer switch on empathy? With psychotherapy she could come to understand her limitations. If Lorri-Jane is going to have a chance to understand what is going on with her family, she needs to slow down. Focusing only on the details of life is not parenting. A maid, a gardener, a cook, a babysitter can take care of the details. Going through life with a single-minded focus on "self" is the ultimate in lack of empathy. Relating to a spouse and children requires an Aspie to turn up the dimmer switch on empathy and take the spotlight off "self."

Zero degrees of empathy

Empathy is the ability to identify with another person's thoughts and feelings AND to respond appropriately. Empathy is recognition of the other. It is identifying with the other. It is responding to another in a way that makes him or her feel understood, appreciated and respected. All of these parts are necessary for *true empathy*. It is not enough to identify and understand the other person: Words are needed, too. Stefan had understood that Adrienne was upset about the cat, but he'd also needed to say something that conveyed his understanding. The same is true for Lorri-Jane. She'd eventually understood that her husband was making toast for the family, not for her; however, she didn't offer an apology that she recognized her error. Both Lorri-Jane and Stefan left their partners and their children feeling misunderstood, abused and rejected.

This extreme lack of empathy is so off-the-chart-low that it doesn't even have a place on the empathy spectrum. It is non-existent. Baron-Cohen refers to it as zero degrees of empathy. *In The Science of Evil: On Empathy and the Origins of Evil,* he writes:

> *Zero degrees of empathy means you have no awareness of how you come across to others, how to interact with others, or how to anticipate their feelings or reactions. Your Empathy Mechanism functions at Level 0. You feel mystified by why relationships don't work out, and your lack of empathy creates a deep-seated self-centeredness. Other people's thoughts and feelings are just off your radar. This leaves you doomed to do your own thing, in your own little bubble, not just oblivious to other people's feelings and thoughts but also oblivious to the idea that there might even be other points of view. The consequence is that you believe 100 percent in the rightness of your own ideas and beliefs, and judge anyone who does not hold your beliefs as wrong or stupid.*

While NTs may experience varying levels of empathy, depending upon circumstances, Aspies are trapped in a world of their own self-focus. The NT can recover from a temporary lapse in empathy, but the Aspie does not know what he or she is missing. From the many examples in this book you can see how zero degrees of empathy results in severely strained interpersonal relationships and a distraught family life.

Zero degrees of empathy is well-portrayed by actor Jesse Eisenberg in the film "The Social Network." Eisenberg's portrayal of Mark Zuckerberg (a co-founder of Facebook, who is sued by the other co-founders) is positively chilling. Zuckerberg doesn't believe he needs to give his full attention to the opposing attorney during his deposition in connection with the lawsuit. Zuckerberg thinks he needs to answer the questions—but not necessarily with respect: Zero degrees of empathy. In another scene, Zuckerberg tries to mend the relationship with his girlfriend by suggesting she just forget his insults and order dinner anyway: Zero degrees of empathy. Even more egregious, Zuckerberg conspires to drive out co-founder, Eduardo Saverin, because the company no longer needs Saverin's money or leadership: More zero degrees of empathy.

Here are a few zero degrees of empathy vignettes from the lives of less famous people.

Joe and Katrina had planned a short trip out of state to attend the wedding of Joe's mother. True, it was going to be her fifth wedding, but Mom had bought tickets for the couple, making the offer very appealing. They'd decided to have a little time away from the kids, welcoming the chance to get away for a mini-vacation. A couple of weeks before the wedding, Katrina's sister was unexpectedly killed in a terrible auto accident. Of course Katrina wanted to scrap the wedding and stay with her sister's family. Not only had she lost a sister, Katrina's children had lost their aunt, and her brother-in-law was in such a state of grief he could hardly function. What had Joe done? He hadn't wanted to waste the airline tickets. And, since he had already arranged the time off work for the vacation, he insisted that Katrina go to the wedding. He reasoned that she'd already had a full two weeks to help out her family, so she could leave to go on the wedding trip: Zero degrees of empathy.

Marilyn, an NT wife and mother of four, was very excited when her Aspie husband, Eddie, agreed to finally spend money on a family vehicle. A van or SUV was what she had been dreaming of for three years. Finally her husband had agreed, and the couple bought a convenient, but fairly luxurious, van with those video screens for the kids in the back seats. Of course Marilyn was surprised when Eddie told her the new van was his to drive to work since they had traded in the vehicle he had been driving. His reasoning was that her car was still in good shape, and he deserved the newer van. Marilyn conceded but asked if Eddie could turn over the van at the end of the work day or on the weekends, so that she could drive the kids to soccer practice and piano lessons. Not exactly what Marilyn had had in mind, but it was an acceptable compromise. The next weekend she decided to use the new van to run the kids to different soccer matches and a birthday party. Imagine her surprise when Marilyn discovered that Eddie had removed all of the seats in the vehicle except for the driver's seat! His reason? Since it was "his" car and he needed lots of space to carry all of his stuff, why bother with passenger seats? Zero degrees of empathy.

Morality and zero degrees of empathy

Zero degrees of empathy can lead to acts of cruelty, make one insensitive to others, or encapsulate the Aspie in social isolation. Zero degrees of empathy does not bode well for long term committed relationships such as co-parenting. Baron-Cohen sums it up well in his book when he writes: "Treating other people as if they were just objects is one of the worst things you can do to another human being, to ignore their subjectivity, their thoughts and feelings."

Baron-Cohen presents some convincing evidence that empathy and morality are different. He refers to those Aspies who lack empathy but have a strong moral code as zero-positive people. Many Aspies have a super-strong moral code that is immovable. An example of this is Marvin, an Aspie and a devout Catholic.

Marvin attends church regularly, sings in the choir and volunteers for many church duties. When Marvin attends a wedding at the church, he always offers to take photographs. In this way he has a reason to talk with people and to move around the crowd. But he is not required to relate empathically. Marvin attends to his responsibilities as a Catholic and enjoys his church community, in part, because it's easy to understand the rules. Many Aspies join a structured church where the rules of moral conduct are spelled out.

There are limits to these Aspie super-moral values. In spite of Marvin's years of devoted service to his church, and the comfort he finds in Catholic dogma, Marvin is lonely. He has yet to find a wife from among the parishioners. One of the reasons is that Marvin is painfully shy and rarely asks a woman out on a date. The other reason? Marvin is looking for a Catholic virgin, because of his super-moral adherence to rigid Catholic values. At age 40, finding a virgin his age may be very hard for Marvin. When I confronted Marvin about this unrealistic goal, he was adamant that, according to biblical Scripture, he must marry a virgin. I countered, stating that it is highly unlikely he'll find a woman his age, who has never been married AND is a virgin. I had a moment of hope that he would adapt when he said it would be acceptable if the woman was divorced. Then he added the caveat that her marriage would have to have been annulled by the Catholic church. (Annulment is the invalidating of a marriage. Generally, annulment is easier if the marriage is unconsummated.) It is useful to remember that within every rigid system there are usually means to accommodate reality.

Zero-positive people compensate for their lack of empathy by adhering to systems of rules. Those with Asperger Syndrome are marvelously adept at systemizing. Their ability to notice and analyze patterns, and figure out how things work is a gift. When change happens in an orderly fashion, there is a pattern that Aspies can discern. The human animal is very adept at noticing patterns, and some of us are better at it than others.

The social world does not have the same regularity of patterns, and this is what throws Aspies. People with Asperger Syndrome are attracted to things such as, overtones in music, the evolution of geological changes in a mountain range, and the types and scale of axles on big rigs—because each is part of a system. As a result of very high levels of systemizing, Aspies with zero degrees of empathy are able to rely on facts and logical analysis to make decisions. If an Aspie has been inculcated with a strong moral code, intent also impacts his or her actions. I will speak more about this concept later in the book.

Out of mind - out of sight

Ending where this chapter began, knowledge is power. Use that power to put a new frame around your relationship. When an Aspie is in the role of spouse and parent, lack of empathy is quite debilitating. As we have seen, Aspies can be rude, clueless, forgetful and even cruel. Lack of empathy can be somewhat offset by the Aspie's good intentions if they have established a strong moral code. At least then the NT co-parent knows what their Aspie believes to be the truth—even if variations of that truth are not allowed. In Aspies, the wiring for empathy is simply nonexistent, and there is no use crying over it. If it is not in the Aspie mind, then it is out of sight.

Instead both the NT and the Aspie need to look to the good intentions behind the clumsy behaviors and bad manners. Co-parents need to be respectful of, kind to, and patient with each other. The Aspie needs to recognize that he or she does indeed have zero degrees of empathy. And, the Aspie needs to stop expecting that his or her grasp of the facts should rule. The NT needs to recognize that zero degrees of empathy can co-exist with feelings of caring. The rules of parenting need to be spelled out. If an AS/NT couple is going to successfully co-parent, both parties need to work with the other's systems.

It might also help to remember there are benefits to having a highly systemized AS co-parent. Your AS husband may do such a marvelous job of wiring the family music system with the most sophisticated sound equipment that it feels like you are in an orchestra pit. Or your AS wife may be a well-paid attorney, because of her exquisite comprehension of a narrow field of law.

On the other hand, your NT wife can be counted upon to navigate an important social event, guiding you all the way, so that you don't have to hide behind a camera to make small talk. Your NT husband may be so kind as to remember all of your relatives' birthdays and even have the perfect gift for each one—wrapped with an appropriate card.

One last reframe before moving on: Remember that children cannot be expected to grasp all that is in this chapter, or the book, for that matter. They need protection and guidance for many years in order to develop healthy adaptations to the unusual stresses in AS/NT homes. They can still respond positively to loving energy demonstrated by their parents. No matter how long it takes, let the children see the two of you willingly talking things out and coming up with mutually agreeable solutions. Then the children will be able to relax in the confident and loving atmosphere you've created. Of course the mutually-agreed-upon solutions should be explicit to all. They may even have to be posted on the refrigerator!

Lessons learned

1. *True empathy* is more than the sum of its parts. *True empathy* is the ability to step into another person's

shoes. It means you can identify and recognize what is going on with another person while at the same time recognizing what is going on with yourself. The third part of *true empathy* is the ability to respond appropriately with words or non-verbal behavior that demonstrate you understand, respect and care for the other person.

2. There are multiple interacting empathy circuits in the brain, creating a spectrum of empathy. These circuits are all so finely tuned that if one is not working, *true empathy* can short-circuit.

3. The empathy spectrum is like a dimmer switch: The degree of empathy experienced at any one time varies. Generally NTs are high on the empathy spectrum, while their AS partners are extremely low.

4. Empathy disorders, such as Asperger Syndrome, are types of psychiatric disorders that are characterized by varying deficits along the empathy spectrum.

5. Baron-Cohen refers to those with Asperger Syndrome as having zero degrees of empathy.

6. Aspies are considered zero-positive people, because they can develop a strong sense of moral conduct, even if they cannot empathize well.

7. Zero degrees of empathy means just that. Zero. Stop expecting something from Aspies that is not wired in. There is freedom in acceptance.

8. Knowledge is power. You now have some understanding about the neurological basis for zero degrees
of empathy in your Aspie co-parent. That provides
you with a place to start creating a pattern of working together for the sake of the family—as long as you
both have loving intentions.

9. Children cannot be expected to utilize the information in this book with the same understanding as
adults. Protect your children from abuse. Give them
lots of unconditional love. Demonstrate that their
parents can negotiate the co-parenting relationship
with patience, respect and love.

CHAPTER SIX

The Rules of Engagement

I have waited until this chapter to introduce the reader to *context blindness*, because it was important to first understand that the parts of the mind/brain are integral to creating meaning from context. Concepts proposed by Smith and Baron-Cohen, such as cognitive empathy, emotional empathy, theory of mind, the spectrum of empathy, empathy circuits, zero degrees of empathy, and so forth—all are part of the holographic array of empathy systems that assist us in creating meaning out of the context. It is the skillful use of context that makes or breaks a relationship. Those with social radar create *true empathy* within the interpersonal context of their lives. Those with empathy disorders create chaotic, and sometimes destructive, meaning from the context.

Peter Vermeulen has proposed *context blindness* to explain Autism Spectrum Disorders (ASDs)[24]. Essentially *context blindness* is the inability of Aspies to distinguish the forest for the trees. Vermeulen defines the opposite of *context blindness* as context sensitivity:

> *Context is what is going on in the environment, outside and inside our brain that influences our way of giving meaning to things. The ability to select elements in the context that are useful and meaningful and to use them is context sensitivity. The neurotypical human brain is, inherently, context sensitive.*[25]

In this chapter, I outline the theory of *context blindness* as it relates to an even broader theory of psychology, developed by Klaus Riegel, dialectical psychology.[26] *Context blindness* profoundly affects the vital process of coming to know ourselves and others. According to Riegel, healthy child development requires successful interrelationships, or dialogues, between people; thus the term "dialectic," or logic and reasoning by dialogue. To carry out such an important task as parenting, more than child care is required. Daycare centers and babysitters can handle childcare, but parenting is so much more. Celebrated family therapist Virginia Satir described parenting as "people making."[27] It is a complex interaction (or dialogue to use Riegel's term), spanning many years and requiring exquisite and empathic communication among mother, father and child. How is this possible when one of the parents is *context blind*?

---

24   Vermeulen, Peter. (2009). *Autism as Context Blindness.* Translated from the Dutch, *Autisme als contextblindheid.* Shawnee Mission, Kansas: Autism Asperger Publishing Company.

25   Vermeulen, Peter. (2009). *Autism as Context Blindness.* Translated from the Dutch, *Autisme als contextblindheid.* Shawnee Mission, Kansas: Autism Asperger Publishing Company: 37

26   Riegel, Klaus. (1979). *Foundations of Dialectical Psychology.* New York: Academic Press.

27   Satir, Virginia (1972). *People Making.* Out of print.

Please don't worry about the academic sound of all this. My goal is to help you apply these theories in a practical way with your Aspie loved ones. I have liberally sprinkled the chapter with examples from real life. I suggest that using the rules of engagement is one way to accommodate the problem of *context blindness*. The rules of engagement offer a template for how to relate without having *true empathy*.

Two Children; Two Contexts

As a daughter of an Aspie who has reared one NT child and one Asperger Syndrome (AS) child, I have countless family stories of *context blindness* versus context sensitivity. The following two anecdotes about my daughters are representative of the dialectic of people making. They demonstrate the differences in how Aspies and NTs understand context. I tell these stories from the perspective of a proud mom with a bit of analysis added by the psychologist part of me.

My youngest daughter, Phoebe, (a neurotypical or NT) was very social right from birth. I swear she smiled within a couple days of first being held in my arms. It hadn't been a surprise when Phoebe asked me if she could attend pre-school along with her older sister, Bianca, who was 5. At the time, Phoebe had been only 2 and in diapers, but I'd made her a deal. The Montessori pre-school required that all children be at least 2½ years old—and toilet trained—before starting school. That was the deal I'd negotiated with Phoebe: She had to be 2½ and be toilet trained, no exceptions. Little Phoebe had agreed to the terms with a proverbial handshake! Her determined and strong-willed personality had insured her success. She'd been ecstatic when she'd achieved her goal and started going to school along with the "big" kids.

Each morning Phoebe would happily get ready for school without any fuss. Her Aspie sister, Bianca, would dawdle and lose track of time while Phoebe was on top of the morning routine. At precisely the time we needed to get into the van and head for Aquinas Montessori School, Phoebe was ready to be strapped into her car seat—and of course wearing her "big girl" panties. We'd made a joy of the morning routine. One part that I'd especially liked was walking Phoebe to her class, giving her a kiss and saying, "Have a nice day Phoebe, and don't wet your panties! Love you."

She would smile back at me with great pride in her accomplishments, both in attending school and being toilet trained. She would give me the thumbs-up gesture with her tiny little hands, and say, "Lo Lu, too, Mommy!" Then she'd run into the classroom, ever so excited to start the daily adventure. I can still see her little ponytail bouncing as she skipped through the door.

In summer later that year, the family had gone along with Daddy to a professional conference where he was to be a presenter. While the girls and I toured the area and played at the hotel pool, Daddy hob knobbed with his colleagues and made ready for his presentation. The day of his speech, Daddy's plan was to leave the hotel room early, get breakfast at the restaurant, and practice his speech before his 8 a.m. start time. Although the girls and I could have slept in, I'd thought it would be nice to give Daddy family support. When he was dressed and ready to leave for breakfast, I told the girls to give Daddy a big hug and kiss and wish him well on delivering his speech. Of course they happily obliged and planted big wet kisses on his cheek.

Then little Phoebe had given Daddy an extra surprise. She'd looked him square in the eye, offered him one of her engaging smiles and confidently pronounced, "Have a nice speech Daddy—and don't wet your panties! Lo Lu." I have to say that Daddy, so impressed by Phoebe's encouragement, used the anecdote to introduce his presentation, much to the amusement of everyone at the seminar.

What better example is there of context sensitivity than this, even if I do say so myself? Little Phoebe had wanted to share love and encouragement with her daddy. She had learned from Mommy how to do that during their interchange every morning at preschool. She'd also been aware that Daddy's speech was momentous, because she had observed him preparing and practicing. She'd wanted to say something that recognized the importance of what he was about to do. She had worked hard to be toilet trained, and Daddy had worked hard for this "speech" moment, too. Perhaps Phoebe had even been aware of how stressful it was to keep her panties dry all morning at preschool—and had wanted to make sure Daddy was prepared for a similar kind of stress at his seminar! But the most important part of Phoebe's message had been the empathic statement that she loved and understood her daddy.

Bianca was no less loving and appreciative of her parents than Phoebe. But she has a very different send-off for her mommy in the following story. Bianca's choice of words has a decidedly Aspie tone. Bianca had been about 8½, and her little sister 5 when I'd packed the car to leave for a week-long stay in Olympia. My plan had been to cloister myself for a week in a hotel in the state capitol and study non-stop for the psychologist licensing exam fast-approaching. I'd put the last of my banker boxes of study materials in the car, then come back into the house for one last hug and kiss goodbye. After that, I'd left the girls upstairs with my secretary, Kathleen, who often doubled as nanny. As I'd opened the car door I'd looked up at the second-story office window. Kathleen had opened the window, so that I could hear the waving children as they excitedly sent me off on my important mission.

Phoebe had sent her daddy off with a few special words that morning in the hotel. Now Bianca had something choice to say to me. "F--- you Mommy. Have a nice day!" (Only she pronounced the whole "F" word.) I'd been speechless. I'd stood there with one foot in the car, holding the door open, my keys in my hand, but I couldn't move. I could only stare in disbelief at Bianca.

Everything was in slow motion as I reeled to comprehend what had just happened. I saw Phoebe take an inquisitive look at her older sister. I saw her make THE decision to speak. To my dismay—yes indeed—I saw Phoebe wave and smile at me; then, imitating Bianca, Phoebe, too, said, "F--- you Mommy. Have a nice day!"

Still unable to speak, I'd looked at Kathleen, who by then had caught her breath and said, "Yes, you heard it correctly. That's what she said."

Of course I had to investigate what on earth was going on. I went back into the house and approached Bianca carefully, because I didn't want her to feel threatened by her faux pas. "Honey," I said, "Where did you learn that expression?" But it was too late, Bianca could tell she had done something wrong. By 8 years of age, Bianca had made enough Aspie blunders to recognize the look of shock and disapproval—especially unpleasant when it came from her mother.

I'd tried to hold my arm around Bianca, giving her reassurance that Mommy loved her, but she'd moved away from my embrace. Defensively she'd said, "But Mommy, it's in your book." And sure enough, it was. Bianca, the self-taught reader, had been browsing my bookshelf for years. Apparently she'd found a book of political cartoons by John Callahan entitled, "Digesting the Child Within and Other Cartoons to Live By."[28] It's actually a reference book I use as a psychotherapist, because Callahan uses cartooning to educate and inspire about those with disabilities. However, the ribald cartoons are definitely not for children.

Bianca had acquired her send-off message from a cartoon entitled, "The Difference Between L.A. and N.Y."[29] In the first frame of the cartoon, a man wearing shorts and standing by a palm tree waves to

28 Callahan, John. (1991). *Digesting the Child Within and Other Cartoons to Live By.* New York: Quill, William Morrow.
29 Callahan, John. (1991). *Digesting the Child Within and Other Cartoons to Live By.* New York: Quill, William Morrow: 53

another man and says, "Have a nice day!" But the "bubble" over his head indicates the real intent of the comment is, "F--- you!" In the second frame of the cartoon, a man wearing an overcoat and carrying a briefcase passes another man on a city street and says, "F--- you!" But the "bubble" over his head shows he really means, "Have a nice day!" Honestly, I have had to explain this cartoon to adults; even so, Bianca had interpreted "F--- you" as a joyful send-off–so why not say it to Mommy!

At first blush, Bianca's amusing mistake appears to be similar to her sister's childish send-off for her daddy. If you take a closer look, you can recognize the *context blindness* in the Mommy send-off. Any parents who have an NT 8 or 9 year old know that by this age children are very familiar with the "F" word and other vulgarities. NT children understand the contextual use of these words and don't dare say them in front of their parents. Aspie youngsters are missing those "brakes."

Bianca was aware that my going was important, and she obviously had a good intention; however, she didn't choose any of a number of appropriate phrases learned from social interaction with her family or friends. She could have said, "Bye-bye, Mommy. Love you." Or she could have said, "Miss you Mommy. Love you." Nope. Instead she chose a phrase she'd learned from a book. Books are like manuals for Bianca. She uses them for instruction just as she'd used "Teen" magazine to try to teach herself about adolescent relationships. This leave-taking scenario demonstrates true *context blindness*.

Human dialogue forms the fabric of our relationships

I hope it is becoming clear how important context is to relationships and how *context blindness* gravely interferes with healthy child rearing. An Aspie may have compassion or love or a good intention, but if he or she cannot express these things in a contextually appropriate way, the meaning is lost and the relationship suffers. Childhood malapropisms and anachronisms can be amusing, but by adulthood they become annoying or worse. For example, what if I'd failed to understand that Bianca meant no harm when she'd said, "F--- you"? What if I'd punished her for using a vulgar term? What if I'd blamed her father for teaching her this term? What if I'd despaired that my child was turning out "badly"? I would have been wrong about these mistaken meanings: I would be in good company. These are the kinds of things that NT parents think when they know nothing of ASD traits.

Context sensitivity is at the center of the dialectic that creates our humanity. We are meant for each other. Without the human social context, we don't have a way to express our unique personalities. Nor do we have the dialectical guidance to develop our life goals. Without context sensitivity, we are alone, and we can become despondent—a feeling that describes many an Aspie as well as their Aspergated loved ones.

Vermeulen describes the history of the term "context" in the quote below. I find it fascinating how appropriately the term applies to the nature of human NT relating. On page 26 of his book, *"Autism as Context Blindness,"* he writes:

> *The term context has its own intriguing historical context. Context comes from the Latin word contextus, the past continuous tense of contextere, which means to 'weave' or 'entwine.' Con means 'inter' and textus means 'woven,' hence the words 'textile' and 'texture,' but also the word text. For the Romans, contextus meant 'connection, strong relationship, interdependence.'*

Think about it. Our human relationships are the weaving together of the meaning of our lives and the lives of our loved ones at this moment in time and across time into a holographic fabric more complex than any tapestry. According to Dialectical Theory, context is constantly being reformatted with each dialogue we have with others. No wonder it is hard for Aspies to track this moving target.

Let's explore this theory a bit further, so that you can apply it to your AS/NT family. According to Riegel, we develop our sense of self from birth, through childhood, adolescence and into adulthood, through a constant interacting with others and the world around us. We make meaning during these interactions and then make meaning of the meaning as we progress through normal developmental stages. Our self concept becomes infused not just with our interpretations of reality, but with how others perceive us and value our being.

Riegel finds that reciprocal relating, or empathizing with each other, is so important to people-making, that his entire theory is named for the concept. The word "dialectical" is related to the phrase "to dialogue" or the ability to converse with others and make meaning of the conversation. In other words, Dialectical Psychology emphasizes the social basis of being human. This message is imparted during the interactive changes in common activities and everyday situations. This complex systems theory has four parts.

1. First, Riegel suggests that in order to understand the human being, one must study a "changing individual in a changing world."

2. Second, there are many developmental progressions, or systems, that an individual is part of at any one time (outer-physical, cultural-sociological, individual-psychological and inner-biological).

3. Third, as these developmental progressions interact, friction is produced that causes conflict, confusion, change, reorganization and growth.

4. Fourth, because human transformation is a product of conflicting developmental progressions, human beings are motivated by discordance and upheaval rather than by stability, equilibrium and rest.

Wow! Does that describe life or what? It is as if we are weaving this tapestry of life, but it keeps morphing with each interpersonal iteration; hence there is never a final product. . . .only more change, more growth, more creative self-expression, more love, more . . . more . . . more.

So can you see why it isn't so easy to put any of us in a neat little box? No two people on the planet have the same fingerprints, and no two people on the planet have the same meaning for everything there is. That's why it is so important to be sensitive to the signals that define the contextual meaning others are making, so that we can relate to them appropriately. NTs have this context sensitivity to one degree or another. Aspies do not. This makes parenting with a partner who has Asperger Syndrome one of the most challenging relationships there is.

Too many windows open leads to context blindness

Aspies are unable to sift through the contextual clues and prioritize them. Baron-Cohen proposes that those with ASD do not have active or working empathy circuits in their brains; however when pressed for contextual information, Aspies often can tell you what they are observing. They just can't tell you which piece of information is vital to making the dialectical connection with their NT loved one. NTs, on the other hand, are able to sift context cues in order to select the one(s) needed to interact and take action in the immediate moment.

Ramon has a clever way of describing the process of the dialectic, which he observes between his mother and grandmother when they argue. I will tell you more about Ramon later in this chapter. For now, know that he is an Aspie teenager, who has learned quite a few social skills because of his mother's devotion to parenting her unusual child. Ramon tells me that often he gets confused in conversations with others or when listening to his mother and grandmother argue, because there are "too many windows open." He explains, "Once you have too many windows open, no matter how many times you click the mouse, your computer just freezes." I never cease to be amazed at how often Aspies use computer metaphors to describe the inner workings of their minds. It's as if they think digitally.

Too many windows are open for Steve when he attends managers' meetings at work. I diagnosed Steve with Asperger Syndrome when he was age 55—when his wife dragged him into therapy one last time to save their marriage. Steve told me that he cannot follow the conversation in a meeting, because the voices all merge into a cacophony of sound (i.e. typical Aspie sensory overload). He relies on a colleague to take notes and debrief him after the meeting.

Too many windows are open for Charlie whenever he is invited to do something he doesn't want to or can't do. He is one of those Aspies who tries to please everyone in order to avoid disappointing them. At 64 he still has not learned how to say "no" graciously. He can easily say "yes" if he is able to accept an invitation, but he can't say "no." Instead, if he is asked to join a friend for dinner, a movie or a glass of wine, and he is unable to attend, Charlie turns and walks away. Or if the invitation comes in an email or text or voicemail, he ignores the message. He doesn't understand that others can accept a polite message declining the offer better than they can accept his ignoring the invitation entirely. Charlie is puzzled that no matter how hard he tries to please, people do not like him.

Too many windows were open for my Uncle Sam when he failed to act compassionately at a critical time. Uncle Sam is my mother's brother. He absolutely stunned me one day when he stopped by the hospital to visit my mother Irene, also an Aspie. My mother was recovering from brain surgery to remove a malignancy. The surgery had been successful at prolonging her life, but we all knew she had only a few months to live. Uncle Sam asked Irene if she would mind taking a private walk with him down the hallway. I thought it very sweet that he asked for this time with his baby sister. I watched as he put his arm around her to help her walk. Before they got out of earshot my Aspie uncle said, "Irene, let's pretend you are not going to die." I noticed my mother pause a moment, then continue walking. Too many windows were open for poor Uncle Sam. He was grief stricken and totally unable to empathize with his sister or the rest of us. Likewise, my poor Aspie mother was probably used to years of this kind of unintended abuse—so she just kept walking.

Too many windows were open for my daughter Bianca when she moved into her own bedroom at age 12. She learned to love this room in the basement with its own private bath, because it was quiet and far away from the hustle and bustle of family life upstairs. In fact she used to call it her "cave." She kept the lights low and her door always shut, so that she had complete privacy from the outside world of people. On her first day in the room, she'd been overwhelmed by all of the changes—even though they were positive ones. We'd carried all of her things in bags and boxes from the room she'd shared with her little sister. After most things were put away, I'd noticed an empty paper grocery bag sitting next to her bed. When I'd reached over to remove it, Bianca had stopped me.

"No!" she'd said and reached for the bag.

"I'm sorry Bianca. Do you need this bag?" I'd offered, handing it to her.

"Yes, I might get sick," she'd explained, as she put the bag back next to her bed.

"Oh aren't you feeling well Honey?" I'd asked.

"No. I am not sick, but I might need the bag if I get sick," she'd explained again.

"Oh, so if you get sick you want the bag?" I'd started to catch her drift.

"Yes, I might not make it to the bathroom," she'd said without a trace of emotion in her voice.

"Okay then. I understand Honey. Are you afraid if you should get sick in your new room you might vomit on your lovely carpet before you get to the bathroom? So you want a paper sack close by just in case," I'd said encouragingly.

Bianca had nodded her head. I'd left the paper sack in her room between her bed and the bathroom where it remained for a few days. Too many windows had been open for Bianca. She'd had no way to prioritize the context for when she might get sick—whether she'd need the bag that day, tomorrow, next week or next month.

What are the rules of engagement?

One method for bridging the gap between *context blind* people and context sensitive people is to have rules of engagement. I get a lot of flak from my NT clients when I suggest this intervention, because they resent having to design rules to live by. They feel like this is "settling" when they'd rather that their Aspie partner develop some empathy and context sensitivity. It is pointless to demand something that your partner is not capable of delivering. Rather, if your Aspie attempts to master the rules of engagement, you can come to accept that their intentions are honorable. Let's see how Consuela and Carmine reconstruct the rules of engagement for their marriage and their family.

Consuela had been blown away when she'd read an email from her estranged husband, Carmine. Carmine had been angry that his wife wanted a divorce. In the same breath that he'd begged her to re-consider, he'd also written, "I am well rid of you parasites!" He'd been referring to his wife and his children. There is just no way to respond to this logic. I always advise my clients to step away from abuse in any form. Consuela agreed with my thinking. Carmine's comments cemented her determination to get a divorce. She hadn't taken his star-tling comment personally though. She was already well aware that her husband's Asperger Syndrome meant that his empathy circuits could not light up.

The real question was how did Carmine get this out of control? He is a successful professional, who travels the world making lots of money for his employer. True, by age 44 he had been married three times and was working on his fourth divorce. Clearly he was not benefitting from the dialectic of social learning. His social skills are limited, and he is known as an overbearing, arrogant know-it-all. Because he is brilliant, Carmine has managed to navigate the corporate ladder to success; the wreckage along the way has been substantial. Beneath that angry exte-rior, Carmine is hurting, and he wants help. That's why he ended up in my office.

On my second appointment with Carmine, I was running late. I'd known I shouldn't have tried carrying my briefcase in one hand, a huge bag of office supplies in the other, my purse slung over one shoulder, a Starbuck's latte in my right hand, and my office keys hanging off my lit-tle finger while navigating the parking lot to the front door of my office building in the rain. It was a recipe for disaster, but I was running late, so I'd taken a chance. I tripped on the last step up to the glass front door, losing my grip on the latte. I watched the lid pop off the paper cup, the drink splash on the glass door, then drop to the step and roll over the edge, spilling the whole cup. Fortunately I hadn't fallen. As I'd leaned forward to recapture my balance, I could see through the glass door that there was a man sitting in the waiting room. It was Carmine, waiting for me to arrive for his appointment.

I wasn't sure if Carmine had seen me drop my coffee and nearly fall "up" the stairs. When I opened the door I got a taste of what Consuela hears on a daily basis. He said, "You know that dyspraxia is a symptom of Asperger's, don' t you?"[30] He looked directly at me with tight lips and piercing eyes. He'd looked malevolent to me (just an example of my NT meaning-making). Obviously he had watched it all and had done nothing to help me.

I took a deep breath. Recognizing the Aspie logic (and the cryptic Aspie sense of humor), I'd said, "Well I suppose you are right. We'll talk about this in our session. Right now, though, I want to put away my things and clean up my mess. Then we can meet." I went to the restroom for paper towels and cleaned up the spilled coffee the best I could. All the while Carmine sat in his chair reading his magazine.

It didn't take long for Carmine and I to get to the subject. (Notice that I ignore the dyspraxia comment for now.) I ask, "Carmine, tell me. What would you have done had it been your wife who had tripped and spilled her coffee?"

Carmine's face lights up (but not his empathy circuits). He says, "Oh! I would have jumped up to help her."

"Why is that?" I ask.

"Well, because she would be real mad at me if I didn't. I've learned that by now," Carmine says emphatically. Carmine understands the rule with his wife but not the empathic reason for the rule. The rule is: She will be angry if he fails to help her.

That was useful information for me. From these comments I knew that Carmine could change. He could at least learn the rules of engagement if not develop *true empathy*. Because Carmine came to me for

---

30   Dyspraxia is a motor coordination problem and a common symptom of those with Asperger Syndrome.

help to save his marriage, and he really believed that I could help, he listened to my next comments.

I patiently offer an explanation to this corporate executive. "Okay Carmine. This is how it works. I am very happy you realize your wife would want your help should she trip and spill a whole Starbuck's grande latte. But here's the rule. In addition to your wife, if any woman trips or drops something, no matter her age, I want you to stand up from your seat and offer to help. Even if she says she is okay, I want you to help. Don't stop offering to help even if she refuses three times. That's the rule."

Carmine looks at me with relief. He says, "That makes sense. It's just that I would feel foolish if I tripped like you did, and I wouldn't want anyone to comment about it. I really want to know the rules of engagement."

I give Carmine a smile. I know that he is getting it. He wants to know the rules of engagement—all such a puzzle to an Aspie. I offer this, "Yes I know that most men may not want the help. They may feel foolish because of all that macho stuff. So the rule is that you can offer help once to a guy and if he refuses, it's okay to let it go. But if a woman trips, I want you to offer to help her at least three times and don't take 'no' for an answer. She really wants your help even if she says 'no.' Does that make sense?" Carmine agrees with a sigh of relief.

One rule doesn't cover everything, but in this case, it is a good start for a man with *context blindness*. Carmine will need to expand his rule book to cover many other interpersonal contingencies.

Let's start when they are young

The dark side of parenting with a partner with Asperger Syndrome is that without education and professional guidance, family life can deteriorate into abuse, severe depression and even suicide. I have been chastised often for taking the position that AS is much more than "neurodiversity," (i.e. the concept that Aspies are just wired differently and that these differences are not problematic to family life).[31] There is hope in understanding the limitations of those with Asperger Syndrome. *Context blindness* doesn't mean that Aspies don't care or have no compassion. It means that they cannot relate unless they are taught the rules of engagement. Ideally this teaching starts in childhood. If it is too late for that, Aspies should be humble enough to learn the rules as adults. They can learn the rules from this book and from their therapists.

Brett, Byron, Drake and Sly are four young men with Asperger Syndrome. All are teenagers in high school. All came to my attention because their respective parents (who do not know each other) wanted help steering their sons back on the track of a secure life plan. Brett had cracked into his parents' online bank account and stolen thousands of dollars. Byron's angry outbursts have erupted into frightening episodes of physical violence that have left holes where he punched the walls with his fists. Drake is a very sweet teen who drowns his sorrows in lone daily marijuana smoking. Sly is a know-it-all who has taken an adversarial approach with his teachers, resulting in numerous school suspensions. His mother has been required to meet with the vice principal, so that Sly can be reinstated in school.

It is not hard to imagine the future of these young men without professional intervention. Their *context blindness* will leave them unprepared for a world where their abusive behaviors will not be allowed—and may even be considered illegal. They may qualify for scholarships to MIT or the University of Michigan. They could have the brilliance to develop the next Microsoft or Facebook or Apple phenomenon. But more than likely they will end up like Carmine, depressed and alone and in danger of losing family. Or worse, they could

---

31   See neurodiversity online at http://en.wikipedia.org/wiki/Neurodiversity.

end up like Gary McKinnon, the Scot who was arrested for spying, because he hacked into the NASA and Pentagon computers looking for evidence that the U.S. government was suppressing information on extra-terrestrial jet propulsion systems.[32]

Just like Carmine, these young Aspies needed to be taught the rules of engagement, so they and their families can survive and thrive. Ramon has an advantage over Brett, Byron, Drake and Sly. Ramon is an exceptional Aspie teenager, because his mother has focused on his training since he was a toddler. She recognized early on that little Ramon was struggling to grasp the nuances of the dialectic of the social world. As a result, his mom sought the help of therapists, educational specialists, and other health care practitioners, who specialize in the treatment of Asperger Syndrome. It has paid off. Ramon is a remarkable young man at age 15. He is on track to graduate from high school with a special education diploma. He has friends, good grades and considerable social skills. Listen to a dialogue with his psychologist.

Ramon usually starts the discussion. "Hi Dr. Kathy. Hey I was wondering if you could help me with a problem I am having with Mom and Grandma?"

"Sure," I say. "Tell me what's going on."

Ramon continues. "Well I know that Mom and Grandma get upset with me when I try to stop them from arguing. I keep trying to tell them to just 'stop it.' But you know they get all upset with me and it turns into a big deal. What am I doing wrong?"

I smile as Ramon asks this innocent question. He trusts me. He trusts psychologists. We have been part of his world since he was a toddler. He views our sessions as meetings with part of his extended family. Doesn't everyone have a psychologist they confide in?

I respond to Ramon's question with sincerity. "Well you know Ramon, your mother and grandmother are NTs, so they may not view

---

32   See Gary McKinnon online. http://en.wikipedia.org/wiki/Gary_McKinnon

their disagreements as being the end of the world the way you view them. They may accept that this is just the way a mother and a daughter discuss things. I know it seems strange, but if you leave them alone, they may actually come to a solution without you."

Ramon looks puzzled. "Well I guess this makes sense, but they really storm through the house when they are arguing, and it is hard for me. I get all fidgety and want to throw things when they get loud."

I give him a look of reassurance and continue. "Good point Ramon. We should talk about how to take care of your feelings when their behavior is upsetting you. But first, are you interested in their NT version of what is going on?" Ramon nods his head, so I continue.

"Women and men are different in the ways they resolve conflict. Men like to get to the facts. Once the facts are understood and accepted, men believe they are on their way to a quick solution. But women want to make sure that everyone has their feelings understood even after a solution is unearthed." I wait for a moment to see if Ramon is following me. He listens and gives me a nod to continue.

"So Ramon, what this means is that your mother and grandmother will continue to hash out the argument a lot longer than it takes to discuss the facts. They may repeat themselves many times before they let it go. They need to make sure that each of them has had a turn to make their feelings known."

Still puzzled, Ramon says."Yea. But how does that help anything?"

I say, "Good question Ramon. Let me explain. We need both kinds of logic in the world. The typical male mind likes to get to the facts and understand the bottom line. The typical female mind wants to make sure that each person gets a chance to express their feelings—and express their acceptance of each other's point of view. It might take a little longer for women to get to an agreement this way, but then everyone feels good about the answer." My explanation is an over-simplification, but when teaching an Aspie youth the rules of engagement, concrete explanations are superior to vague generalities.

Ramon brightens as he grasps the concept. He asks, "Is this why more males like to work with tools and more females like to work with people?"

I laugh out loud and smile broadly when I hear Ramon's evaluation of gender differences. He has found a rule to expand his dialectical context. "Yes," I say. "I think you've got it Ramon. So do you think you can let the women in your life resolve problems without interfering even if it appears they are taking forever?"

Ramon shakes his head with a look on his face of bemused acceptance. He says, "Yea I guess I will have to let my NT wife do it that way when I get married." It is so refreshing to hear Ramon say these things. He has figured out a lot about the NT world and assumes that he will have an NT wife one day. Given the odds—and his expanding rules of engagement repertoire—he is probably correct.

Connecting through plug-ins

Marilyn looked at me with tears in her eyes and said, "I don't know if I can live like this forever. I know my husband is a good man, but even though he is learning the rules of engagement, as you call them, he is still not capable of really connecting with me. He doesn't really empathize with me. Although he tries real hard, he doesn't really know what is in my heart. And he doesn't seem to miss not knowing. When we are done talking, he just walks away, leaving me to take care of all of the feelings in the family including my own. Will this ever change?"

Answering Marilyn's question is the purpose of this book. The bottom line for an NT co-parenting with an Aspie partner is that learning the rules of engagement is not the same as developing context sensitivity and *true empathy*. Without empathy your Aspie partner and Aspie children will not relate to you, the NT, in the way your context sensitivity wants. Without empathy, Aspies can't sort through the contextual clues and assess which ones to address and in which order of priority. You probably won't feel the "connection" that so many NTs crave in their interactions with their AS loved ones. All you can do is know that you are loved by how much work your Aspie is willing to put into the relationship.

Adrienne feels fortunate that her AS husband, Stefan, is willing to put in the work. If you recall I introduced you to this couple in the chapter, "Out of Brain - Out of Mind." Stefan made the off-hand comment to Adrienne about the cat that sent her into a tirade about how uncaring he is. The couple was able to work out this problem in therapy but they have been doing more than just working out one disagreement at a time. They have been practicing the rules of engagement for a variety of situations, and inventing new rules that suit them and their family. Because Stefan is motivated to do the right thing by his wife and children, Adrienne feels more loved even without an empathic connection. Adrienne's dialectical context has expanded to include the rules of engagement as a means to connect with her husband. This is a remarkable reframe.

At one session with the couple, I'd noticed a change in Stefan. Instead of walking into the office ahead of his wife and grabbing his favorite chair, Stefan had paused at the door and allowed Adrienne to enter first. He'd waited for her to sit down, then he'd done so. This little bit of gentlemanly effort had seemed to please Adrienne, who'd smiled broadly at her husband when he'd looked in her direction. I'd smiled too and said, "Stefan I have noticed a change in you lately. You seem happier. What do you think is going on?"

Before Stefan can speak Adrienne interrupts with a chuckle. "Yes, one change is that he allowed me to come through the door first, without bumping me out of the way, and he even let me pick my chair.

That's very nice. Thank you." Obviously Stefan has learned an important rule of engagement, a simple bit of gentlemanly politeness that means so much to Adrienne.

Stefan smiles a mischievous grin and explains his thinking on what is different. "Well Dr. Marshack, I figured out something about my *context blindness*. I know I am not any good at reading Adrienne or figuring out which piece of the context I should focus on, but if I slow down and try to get to the other side of my brain, I come up with a better approach. I just can't say or do the first thing that pops into my head. It might be all wrong."

I nod with approval and Stefan continues by offering a computer metaphor. "Dr. Marshack, do you know what threads are? Or maybe a better way to look at it is like subroutines [sequences of computer instructions that can be used repeatedly] in a computer program. Anyway, I figure that I need to have a politeness checker running in the background of my mind to remind me to be a gentleman."

> "I know I am not any good at . . . figuring out which piece of the context I should focus on, but if I slow down and try to get to the other side of my brain, I come up with a better approach. I just can't say or do the first thing that pops into my head. It might be all wrong. . . . Anyway, I figure that I need to have a 'politeness checker' running in the background of my mind to remind me to be a gentleman."

Adrienne and I are very amused by the metaphor and lean forward to hear more about Stefan's new "software" for his brain. Stefan continues, "Then I can just download plug-ins [small pieces of software that supplement a larger program] whenever there is a new social skill I have to learn. The plug-in can work with my politeness checker to keep me on track in the conversation with Adrienne."

With that explanation Stefan smiles at both of us. I sense the pleasure he feels about his clever analysis. We are all pleased—very. Obviously Stefan has discovered tools to convey to his wife that she is loved and appreciated. This feels like reciprocal caring to Adrienne, even if it is not *true empathy.*

Tips for Creating rules of engagement

Since we are all "changing individuals in a changing world" there is not a one-size-fits-all approach to the rules of engagement. The rules need to be fashioned to fit each family specifically. Each AS/NT parenting couple will have a range of context sensitivity to work with. Imagine the complications when you are designing rules to include adults and children with a complex range of abilities. The rules of engagement aren't really hard and fast rules. Like a computer program, rules of engagement have room for upgrades. Plus, you may be surprised to find that your rules "software" creates unexpected solutions.

It is for this reason that I have taken the time to introduce you to Dialectical Psychology and its components: theory of mind, empathy disorders, empathy imbalance hypothesis and *context blindness.* With this theoretical model, you can design your own personalized rules of engagement and "morph" them as the need arises. For starters, I have listed four basic rules of engagement that should be used by every AS/NT parenting couple.

Rule No 1. Change the environment to make it more AS/NT friendly

The very first rule you should consider is: Change the environment to make it more AS/NT friendly. I won't go into detail, but there are dozens of resources to help you accomplish this (see the AAPC bookstore at www.aapc.com). For example, if your Aspie has sensory sensitivities, don't overwhelm them. Reduce the sound, sight, smell and tactile overload. Or you can create a "cave" away from the hustle-bustle of the family for those Aspies who wear out easily from socializing.

Likewise you need to create an environment that is friendly for the NTs. If you can afford it, hire help for housework and lawn care to save energy for the emotional work NTs must do to support their Aspies. Some AS/NT couples even rent a city apartment where one parent at a time can make a break for it. There are many options for creating an AS/NT friendly environment for your family. I suggest several in this book. The essence is to think of your family's needs first and to stop worrying about fitting in with the dominant culture.

Rule No. 2. Build your team

Obviously you need to build a team of professionals and supportive friends and family to help you parent. I highly recommend that in addition to your psychologist, special education teachers, speech pathologist, naturopath, pediatrician and daycare provider, you find a good support group. I offer such a group for NTs in Portland, Oregon, and online for worldwide members at http://www.meetup.com/Asperger-Syndrome-Partners-Family-of-Adults-with-ASD/. There are also a number of support and social groups for Aspies, parents, partners and children on the spectrum. Try checking the Internet for groups in your area that may be associated with your local autism society. A good team can offer emotional and physical support as well as ideas for building your rules of engagement.

Rule No. 3. Carry a notebook

Stefan has learned to carry a notebook with him to jot down the rules of engagement as they come up in his life with Adrienne and the children. He and Adrienne review his notes from time to time to clarify the rules. Without the notebook, the Aspie parent is very likely to forget the interpersonal lesson because of his or her *context blindness.* This is a very important rule if the members of an AS/NT parenting team are to build successful rapport. For example, one day Stefan used his notebook to clarify a very important rule of the dialectic of relationships. We were discussing the validity of social media, such as Facebook. He complained that he thought Facebook was a waste of time and only served to allow people to gossip and spy on others. I challenged his reasoning

"Stefan, isn't it true that you like donuts?" I ask.

"Yes I do. In fact I like this one shop near your office. I stop in to buy a donut whenever I come to our appointments," Stefan replies.

"Well I believe that donuts are unnecessary and even harmful to your health. They are full of empty calories. Further they load your system with sugar and fat. No. I don't believe in donuts at all," I say emphatically.

Stefan looks at me curiously as it dawns on him that I am up to something. Then he counters with a grin, "But I like donuts anyway."

"Precisely," I say. "You eat donuts because they are fun. Donuts bring you pleasure, just as Facebook brings pleasure to those who use it."

Before I can explain more, Stefan pulls out his notebook and says, "Just a minute. Let me write this down. Donuts equal Pleasure. Facebook equals Pleasure. So the new rule is that Donuts equal Facebook. Ha!" Stefan is obviously enthused about his discovery.

I add my explanation. "You got it Stefan. Please don't judge another person's pleasure just because you don't like it. Remember, donuts are really worthless food, but they are fun. Don't you think we all need more fun and pleasure in our lives?"

"Yes indeed Dr. Marshack," Stefan affirms. "I will try to notice other people's donuts, so that I don't step on their fun."

Rule No. 4. Say, "That's right"

This is one of my all-time favorite rules for NTs, because it helps to pull the brain out of a stuck place. Whenever anyone confuses you with a comment or a behavior, you can say to yourself, "That's right." Those words will trigger a message like Stefan's donut rule does for him. In other words, you are acknowledging the other person is doing or saying something with good intention. You may not understand their intention, but it makes sense to them, and you are honoring this. It is just as "right" for them as any of your beliefs and behaviors are for you. Once you stop judging the other person, you can start the process of understanding and problem solving—from a neutral, or even loving, place. This is a wonderful gift to give your AS partner and children.

I have to acknowledge that this last rule, saying, "That's right," is a bit more complex than the typical rules of engagement. It actually requires empathy to carry it off well, which is why I reserve this rule for the NT parent/partner. This rule requires an appreciation of the underlying intentions of the other person: That requires a great deal of skill and emotional balance. I discuss the important concept of intention further in the coming chapter, "Power of Intention."

Now it's your turn to design your own rules of engagement in order to deal with the myriad of relationship problems that crop up each day in your AS/NT parenting partnership. Perhaps you want to incorporate the Ten Commandments into your rules, or the universal Golden

Rule, which is to treat others as you would like them to treat you. One popular rule of engagement is, when asked a question, to never say, "No," until you have waited 20 to 30 minutes to really think about it. Another rule is to use the "One-to-Five Scale." This is a system that works well to regulate emotions by rating emotional responses. You can create rules that will help your Aspies understand when to: raise their voice; interrupt an adult; or laugh loudly. If you need help with any of these rules, please check out the AAPC bookstore online.

The dark side of the moon

Dialectical Psychology gives us a new way to look at empathy disorders, such as Asperger Syndrome. Because Aspies miss out on the normal dialectic of human development that is so vital, they struggle in their roles as parent and partner. I hope this chapter has helped you to better understand the work cut out for AS/NT co-parents. A child's healthy growth depends upon developing a strong sense of self—something that accrues over the years as a result of relating to their parents and others with *true empathy*. People-making takes a great deal more effort than teaching simple concrete life skills, such as how to read or make a bed. The most important learning from childhood is to gain the sense of being understood and valued by others, especially by parents. With this level of confidence in oneself, a child can go on to master many, many life skills on his or her own.

Context blindness is like the dark side of the moon where the sun never shines. It just isn't possible to expect a truly empathic response from someone with Asperger Syndrome. They don't have the empathy circuits to distinguish the emotions and meaning when relating to their loved ones. Nor do they have the ability to act appropriately to context. We see in this book how out of control family life can get when an Aspie's *context blindness* is left untreated. If the Aspie parent is willing to learn alternative methods of relating and can negotiate the rules of engagement with the NT spouse/partner, then he or she may be able to convey the love and appreciation that their children need to develop a healthy sense of self-esteem. It's not the same as a truly empathic connection, the kind of connection felt instantly in the heart. But it is another kind of love. After all, love is what's at the center of the parent/child relationship.

Lessons learned

1. People-making is the most important job of parenting. It requires that a child develop a strong sense of self in order to grow into a healthy, independent adult.

2. Dialectical Psychology is the concept that we come to know ourselves in relationship to others.

3. A child's sense of self can best be nurtured through empathic human relating, first with parents and eventually with others.

4. When a parent has Asperger Syndrome, he or she has an empathy disorder. In particular they have *context blindness*, which leaves them ill equipped to understand the minds and actions of others.

5. Without proper psychological treatment and education, a parent with Asperger Syndrome may contribute to a destructive home environment. AS/NT

parents should always seek the help of a trained psychologist or mental health professional.

6. While parents with Asperger Syndrome cannot learn empathy, they can learn the rules of engagement. Seek out therapists and educators who teach these rules, so that your Aspie loved ones get help.

7. We are "changing individuals in a changing world." Therefore the rules of engagement need to "morph" with Aspies and NTs in the context of their changing AS/NT families.

8. Many parents and partners with Asperger Syndrome refuse to seek help. It is one thing to cling to the idea that Aspies are just different, as held in the concept of neurodiversity. It is quite another to leave a child struggling to relate to an emotionally unavailable Aspie parent. Get professional help for the child even if the Aspie parent refuses help.

9. Love is still love, and it is the center of the parent/child relationship. If the Aspie parent cannot give a truly empathic heart connection, he or she can still offer love. It's love of another kind. It's a love demonstrated through loving intention, using techniques from the rules of engagement.

CHAPTER SEVEN

Hapa Aspie

Parenting children in a home with an Aspie parent is very complex, particularly if you have Aspie and neurotypical (NT) children. In the first three chapters, I described the chaos of these families and the ensuing distress that NTs feel in this environment. In the second three chapters, I outlined: theories to help you better understand why Aspies do what they do; and how to change the negative outcome with the rules of engagement. In the remaining four chapters, I answer specific questions about how to resolve more complex and unique problems that arise when you are parenting with a partner or spouse with Asperger Syndrome. We do need more than the rules of engagement to rectify these problems.

Within the dialectic of interacting with a *context blind* Aspie partner, the context sensitive NT spouse has to switch back and forth between the worlds of Aspie partner, Aspie children and NT children. This is also true for NT children. Their world is a very confusing mix. At school or with friends, they can engage in the NT dialectic that reinforces their perception of reality. At home, they get mixed signals. It is hard for adults to maneuver the unusual world of Aspie/NT family life: Imagine how hard it is for NT children.

In this chapter, I discuss how NT children respond to these mixed signals. During crucial developmental stages, NT children who get different signals from their parents and their siblings learn to cope in unique ways that last a lifetime. Very often, NT children are lonely, depressed and feel invisible to others. They frequently develop a variety of Aspie-like traits, too. That's not surprising, given that's what is modeled for them. One of my NT partners' support group members defined this phenomenon as "Aspergated," or being Aspie-like by association. I prefer the term "Hapa Aspie," which is derived from the Hawaiian slang word, "Hapa," meaning half. For children who are NT growing up in an Asperger/NT family, I think that Hapa Aspie fits. Whether by genetic inheritance or behavioral learning, NT children from these families acquire a unique perspective that can best be explained as Hapa Aspie.

Stuck between "No" and "Yes"

In the early days of parenting an NT younger child and an AS older one, I marveled at their delightful differences. I enjoyed mothering my daughters then. I had no idea what was ahead for either of them—or me—as the Asperger element gained a hold on us. As most parents do, I learned a lot about myself from my children, because for NTs these relationships are reciprocal. Only when I discovered my mother had Asperger Syndrome did I realize my own Hapa Aspie nature. It had been an exciting and painfully depressing realization: Exciting because knowledge is power; depressing because of all the years lost and the relationships marred. I have worked all of my life to free myself from my mother's emotional oppression. Yet, I still carry with me the shaping from those baby years—when Mother could not connect with me. She'd looked into my eyes and seen a child, but she hadn't seen me.

One day when I was 13, my mother and I had an argument. I hadn't misbehaved. She hadn't been furious and screaming at me in one of her rages over some childish infraction of the rules. This had been different. We'd had a disagreement about something I can't even remember anymore. I'd explained my point of view, and my mother had continued to challenge my position with her laser-like logic. When it came to a disagreement with my mother, there was ever only one answer. Because of her mind-blindness, the only correct answer was hers. She would not give me an inch. Out of desperation I'd looked her square in the eye and bravely confronted this formidable authority figure. I'd pleaded, "Mom! Isn't it possible that we just think differently?"

No response. My innocent, yet insightful, question had stopped her in her tracks. I can still see her standing there in the open doorway between the kitchen and the living room, the light from the fixture over the kitchen table shining behind her body and framing her in a harsh glare. Her almond-shaped eyes had widened into round saucers, and she'd stared at me—just stared at me—with the vacant look she'd get when her mind would go blank (a look typical of Aspies). Time had stood still as I'd waited for a response. Nothing. Nothing. Nothing. Calm as a cucumber, with not a trace of anger remaining, she'd slowly turned around and gone into the kitchen where she'd lit a cigarette and poured herself a cup of coffee.

That was it? Nothing? Had I won the argument? Had she understand my point of view? Had she still disagreed but just given up? She'd given no hint. She'd just walked away as if I hadn't existed. It was as if my incomprehensible question had crashed her central processing unit. There was the disconnect again. My mother's mind-blindness hadn't been able to process that her daughter had a mind at all, let alone that we thought differently.

My NT Dad had been different, and I'd relished discussions with him. He'd smiled at me as I'd worked my childish logic against his mature wisdom. He'd acknowledged that I had a good point or two even if he disagreed with me. He'd never just quit. He'd never grilled me. He hadn't taken me on like I was an opponent. Instead he'd shown me respect and love that I could feel—in my heart. I'd never felt that from my mother. Sometimes Dad would concede to me. Sometimes I would concede to him. It was a reciprocal relationship, and we thoroughly enjoyed each other's company—even when we disagreed.

One of my most cherished moments with Dad is an argument we had when I was 26 or 27. By then we'd argued about politics and religion and philosophy and women's rights. Sometimes I'd cried, because I felt so passionately about things. I'd never felt he wasn't listening. On this one particular day, Dad had stopped mid-argument, looked lovingly at me and, with pride in his voice, said, "I love having a daughter who knows things I don't know!" Then we'd hugged. I'll never forget that moment for the rest of my life. He'd recognized ME, his grown child with her own perceptions of reality. What a stark contrast to the unforgettable moment with Mother when I'd been 13 and had wanted her approval, too.

In my mind, I like to replay that argument with my mother as if she'd had NT comprehension. I can imagine her looking at me, smiling, and answering my question with a more appropriate motherly comment such as, "Well now, I guess I never thought of that. You do have a mind of your own don't you? You are not a little girl anymore, and you are smart enough to teach your mother a thing or two!" But that didn't happen. She never, ever said those words. Instead, my mother, my primary nurturing parent, left me with a lifetime of being stuck between saying, "No," and saying, "Yes." There has been no in-between in my personal world of loving relationships. If someone is the least bit reserved, I shut down and move away. If they don't respond to my first offer, I expect rejection and quit. In order to reach beyond my defenses to the authentic me, people need to be so gregarious that I can't refuse—or so obtuse that they don't recognize my reluctance to engage. This is really a sad state of affairs, but very like a Hapa Aspie.

Jason needs his own therapist

Helen sits with her head in her hands, beside herself with grief over the latest Grant story. "Dr. Marshack. What am I supposed to do? I can't monitor Grant's relationship with the children anymore. These may seem like little things, but I fear that they are marring the kids for life. Am I over-reacting?"

"Helen," I say, "By now you know that I believe you, and I believe in your good judgment. You are not over-reacting to be concerned about Grant's interactions with the children. Because of his Asperger Syndrome and his lack of empathy and *context blindness*, he can really confuse your children. This confusion can persist for a lifetime. When kids are young, they don't always analyze everything. They just absorb it and create a belief about it. Tell me what happened, and we will figure out what you can do to help your children." Helen explains.

We went to Sunday breakfast at a restaurant last week. Before we got out of the car Grant reminded the kids that they couldn't order more than $7.50 each from the menu. He has this rigid belief about money, and you can't reason with him. Plus the kids are not little anymore. They are 15. Good grief, Jason is taller than me and almost as tall as his father. The twins can't order from the kids' menu. But Grant gets livid if the kids even ask for anything costing more than $7.50.

Helen hesitates and looks at me for approval since she can't shake the belief that she is over-reacting. I give her a smile and nod for her to continue.

We are seated at our table when Grant decides to go to the restroom. He tells me what he wants to order from the menu—always more than $7.50, then gives me instructions to order for him when the wait person arrives. While he is gone, Jason asks if he can order a side of sausage links to his main course, which would boost his total over $7.50. I approved the choice—because he offered to share the sausage with his sister—even though this brought his total to $10.50.

When Grant came back to the table he was in a good mood. His food was served shortly and we all chatted happily for a change. Until the bill came. When Grant saw that Jason had ordered more than $7.50 he was furious. When I tried to explain that I had authorized it, Grant came unglued. Right there in the restaurant. He called me a liar. Worse, he demanded that Jason pay him back for the extra money he had spent. Oh Dr. Marshack, it is impossible to save the children from this kind of insanity. What should I do?

I respond, "Helen, these are the same kinds of problems that others face who co-parent with an Aspie partner. I could explain to you all of the reasons that Grant gets stuck in his own reasoning. You know that he has a heightened sense of justice and that's why he felt you betrayed him over sausage links. You know that he thinks of the children as if they are extensions of him rather than unique individuals; hence he cannot comprehend how much food they might need to eat now that they are older. I could explain all of this to you all over again, but you and I both know an explanation will not help. Insight into Asperger's is not enough. You need an action plan to rescue your children from this mental abuse."

Helen has a wide-eyed look of relief on her face. The alarm over her children's mental health and self-esteem has been growing steadily over the last year—since she'd faced her husband's Asperger Syndrome. She is feeling the pressure to help them but is at a loss as to what to do.

Thank you, Dr. Marshack, for calling it 'abuse.' I need your perspective. Please let me tell you more before I burst. I know you understand, but I also need to talk about these things. To actually be free to complain about Grant is so important to me, because he won't listen.

Helen looks at me again. This time it's a look of gratitude, not a look seeking permission to speak. She continues.

It is bad enough that Grant made this scene in the restaurant, but he continued the raging when we got home. He stood by Jason's door—demanding, demanding, demanding—until Jason gave him the extra $3 he supposedly owed his dad for breakfast. Then Grant went into the kitchen and blew up again. He'd determined that Jason had failed to clean the kitchen properly the night before. He screamed so loudly I was sure the neighbors could hear. And Grant doesn't just scream: He called Jason every name in the book. I was terrified when he stomped back to Jason's room with a frying pan in his hand. I didn't know if he was going to hit Jason with it or what. Do you know what he did Dr. Marshack?

I twist nervously in my seat, wondering if I will have to make a child abuse report. "Tell me Helen," I say warily, "What did Grant do?"

Grant was so crazed, that he demanded Jason pay him $20 for the frying pan, because it had a scratch in the Teflon coating. He blamed Jason for being careless with washing the frying pan. When I heard this accusation, I just couldn't stand it anymore. I stormed down the hallway, grabbed the frying pan out of Grant's hands and told him to 'Shut up!' Grant tried to yell back at me, but I told him, 'Just keep it up, and I'll smack you with this pan. Now get out of my face and go to your room!' Really Dr. Marshack, I said all of that—like I was scolding a child and sending him to time out. Grant did exactly as I told him to do. We didn't see him for the rest of the day.

The tension in my shoulders eases. At least I don't have to make a child abuse report, and I don't have to worry that Helen is going to be arrested again (such as the unfortunate time she was arrested last year when she tried to protect Jason from Grant and broke Grant's glasses). However, the possibility of violence in this home is growing again, and Helen needs a better plan. Helen needs an emergency plan to help protect herself and her children in the moment.[33] She also needs a long-term plan to resolve the emotional damage that Grant is doing to his NT child. But before I can open my mouth to explain these plans,

---

33   Normally when a client faces the possibility of serious physical abuse I suggest an emergency plan that will keep them and their children safe. For example, I suggest that they pack a bag with clothing and overnight essentials for both the parent and their children and either keep it in the car or with a close friend or relative in case they have to make a quick departure.

Helen interrupts. She so desperately needs to tell her story that I let her go on.

"There's more Dr. Marshack. There's more. Grant is just so incompetent as a parent that the kids hate him some days. I know they love him, too, but he abuses and confuses them. Yesterday he scolded Jason for slipping his shoes on and off without lacing them. You know how the kids are these days. They have this weird way of tying the laces under the tongue so that all they have to do is slip the shoes on or off. The shoes look laced up, sort of. So Grant forced Jason to sit down, pull the laces out of his shoes, re-lace them, then tie them on the top of the shoe before he could leave the house. Jason was humiliated, but that's not the end. Once Jason was out the door, Grant slipped on his own shoes—without lacing them— and followed Jason to the car. Honestly, Grant scolded Jason for putting on his shoes the same way that Grant does. What's up with that?"

Helen gave me that Mona Lisa smile I have seen so often. I think her distress is lessened if she can laugh at the way Grant makes himself a fool with these contradictions. Helen's smile is my cue that I can say something now. "Helen, I think it is long overdue for Jason to have his own psychologist. Jasmine sees a therapist to help her with problems associated with her Asperger Syndrome, such as social skills and emotional regulation. You have me. But Jason only has you and that is not enough. He needs his own therapist to confide in. That way he won't feel caught in the middle of his parents. Does this make sense?" I look at Helen to see if she is following me. She is tearful.

I continue, "I know you hoped that Jason would not be harmed by his father's and sister's inconsistencies and abusiveness, but he is being harmed. I know you hoped that your love for him and your solid mothering would take care of everything, but you are not enough. Jason is torn between his parents, trapped between the worlds of the Aspie and the NT. While he is clearly NT, he wants his father's love and wants to please him. As long as you and Grant are at odds with each other, Jason, and Jasmine, for that matter, does not have a choice. If they choose you, then they have to reject their father. If they choose Dad, they have to reject you. Don't put them in that position. Give Jason another person who can help him and who has no family agenda. With his therapist he has a chance to solve these problems now, rather than grow up to be Hapa Aspie, or half Aspie and half NT, but not really either. Are you following me?"

Helen nods her head and wipes away her tears. She had hoped that Jason would be protected from his father's lack of empathy and self absorption, but it is not to be.

I know you are right Dr. Marshack. But I am so angry that Grant has caused this. I know he has a disability, but why do the kids have to pay the price? Oh I know you can't answer that question. It is Grant who needs therapy, you know, but he tells me he is just fine. In his narrow little world, occupied by a population of one, I suppose he doesn't need help. He is just fine with no meaningful relationships!

Anger and tears for Helen. This is a good sign that she is letting go of her hold on "helicoptering," or having to solve everything herself. She needs to build a team of others who can help parent when she and Grant can't.

At age 6 we start to reason

The truth is that Jason should have been in therapy long before his 15th birthday to halt the development of his Hapa Aspie nature. By 15 Jason has already developed his basic social skills, his perspective on the world, and his belief about who he is in relation to others. It will take a bit of work in therapy to reorganize these beliefs and to allow Jason's authentic self to emerge from the chaos of feeling torn between the Aspie world and the NT world.

By age 6, children start to make a marvelous change from being self-absorbed babies to being more reasonable people. That's why they can learn to stand in line facing the teacher, or learn to raise their hand to get a drink of water. Besides being the time for getting permanent teeth, growing bones and learning to follow a teacher's commands, this is a period of profound social awareness. The all-important theory of mind arises. In other words, 6 year olds develop the awareness that other people have minds, plans and desires of their own. Children at this age want to learn the social rules of their group and community. This is when they start forming their friendship groups, usually divided along gender lines. They also start tuning in to the concepts of fairness and justice. They may complain if one person takes more than their share of food or parental time.

What is responsible for this change? In large part it is due to a process called adrenarche, when signals from the pituitary gland tell the adrenal glands to start a cascade of hormonal changes. Some adrenal hormones, such as dihydroepiandrosterone (DHEA), are potent anti-oxidants and protect the health of the child's brain neurons. Adrenal hormones divert glucose in the brain to foster the maturation of the insula and anterior cingulate cortex, brain regions vital to interpreting social and emotional cues. In other words, by middle childhood, the brain is open to learning from the social cues of others.

But what happens to the NT 6-year-old boy who is sandwiched between an Asperger sister and an Asperger father, and who is helicoptered over by his NT mother? This child has a lot to contend with. How does a child of 6 make sense of the fact that he has a theory of mind (and context sensitivity) but his Aspie father doesn't? How does the NT child connect with his Aspie sister when she is not the least interested in developing a friendship network at school like all of the other children? How does the NT child develop a sense of self in relationship to his mother when Mom is at odds with Dad? Is he, like his mother, supposed to be conflicted about his father? Or does the NT child feel like a failure, because he cannot resolve the parental conflict?

I remember being 6 and going through this important transition. I loved first grade. My teacher was Mrs. Alderson, a warm and grandmotherly woman who used colored chalk on the blackboard. There was time for play, and there was time for work. Mrs. Alderson always had a twinkle in her eye. If we students were very, very good, Mrs. Alderson would allow us to play in the kindergarten room after the kindergarten children had left for the day. Mrs. Alderson understood that while we were responsible first graders, we also needed to hang onto those baby years a little bit longer and play with TinkerToys.

By second grade, something had changed in my life. I suspect that, like Jason, I'd become aware that my Asperger parent was, well, not aware of me: Not in the way that Mrs. Alderson was aware of me. I'd been happy and outgoing in first grade, but I'd developed into a frightened, lonely little girl in second grade. I'd decided to do something about it. With my newly developing theory of mind and social awareness, I'd concocted a plot to get my mother's attention. I'd pretended to have trouble in reading group. I was a good reader by then and placed in the top reading group. What better way to get the attention of my sweet teacher, Mrs. Bellerby, than by faltering over the words as I read aloud from our second-grade reader. It worked! Mrs. Bellerby had called my mother for a conference at school to discuss how to help little Kathy improve her reading.

At age 7, I'd figured out that one way to get my mother's attention was to have a problem at school. Secondly I'd picked Mother's favorite subject, reading. My Aspie mother loved to read. She would read all the way through dinner and into the wee hours of the morning. She would ignore her children when we came home from school, forgo cooking dinner, and not notice when we tucked ourselves into bed, all because she was reading.

When my mother found out from Mrs. Bellerby that I was struggling with reading, she took it very seriously. She began reading with me every night, but I don't remember any joy in this time together. Mother was trying to be a good parent. She'd wanted to help her daughter with a problem, but reading wasn't my problem. Mother was my problem; or rather the absence of a loving connection was the problem. One grading period, Mrs. Bellerby noted on my report card that I had made miraculous strides in reading and was once again in the top reading group. Thinking the goal was accomplished, my mother stopped reading with me.

I was a youngster, yet I'd already figured out a bit about my mother. Sadly, I'd also developed a belief that it was my responsibility to create a way to connect with her. Failing time and again to connect with my mother, I'd come to believe that my mother didn't really love me—because I was not lovable. That's how children think; that it is their fault. Sad. I had known that Dad loved me. But, like Jason, I'd known my parents were in constant conflict; thus neither of them had been available to me. Very sad.

Two halves do not make a whole

I firmly believe that NT children growing up with an Aspie parent should have their own therapist and from a very early age. These children are exposed to mind-bending logic that is akin to brain-washing. It is easy to destroy the confidence of a child with inconsistent parenting. It is easy to confuse the child about their sense of reality by placing them in illogical conundrums. It is not enough to have a loving parent who can model the NT reality for the child: When the child is caught between two authority figures and loves and depends on both, additional help is needed for that struggling child. A soccer coach can inspire the child. A camp counselor can be a buddy. A kind teacher is there for only one year. NT children need more than a few temporary, albeit caring role models. NT children in these families need a long-term relationship with a psychologist, who can model a healthy reciprocal relationship and help the child build the skills needed to navigate the tense world of AS/NT relationships. Otherwise, the child will grow up to be Hapa Aspie—half NT and half Aspie—two halves that do not make a whole. There is always something missing, and the child feels this lack of integration keenly.

My Hapa Aspie world view is always partitioned into two parts, and this started a long time ago as a result of my AS/NT parents' modeling. It's not quite the black-and-white thinking of the Aspie, but it's certainly divided into two extreme polarities. Notice in this chapter that I refer to "my mother" and "Dad." Even my language reflects this emotional dichotomy. I feel very little connection with "my mother" (lower case "m"). I feel a vibrant loving interaction with "Dad," (upper case "D") even though he has passed away. I have noticed this with other Hapa Aspies, too, even the children. Just think about the world view of a Hapa Aspie who divides their life this way. Like a light switch, sometimes our relationships are turned on, and sometimes they are turned

My Hapa Aspie world view is always partitioned into two parts, and this started a long time ago as a result of my AS/NT parents' modeling. It's not quite the black-and-white thinking of the Aspie, but it's certainly divided into two extreme polarities. . . .Like a light switch, sometimes our relationships are turned on, and sometimes they are turned off, but there is no in-between, no adjusting with a dimmer switch.

off, but there is no in-between, no adjusting with a dimmer switch.

Helen is coming to terms with her own Hapa Aspie nature. I have always felt that she and I have far more in common than we know. One day she shares this story with me.

"Dr. Marshack, I always thought that Jasmine inherited her Asperger Syndrome from Grant, but now I wonder how many of my relatives might be on the Autism Spectrum."

I am very curious and encourage Helen. "Really Helen? Please tell me more about this. What are you thinking?" Helen continues.

Well I don't think Mom is an Aspie, but I do wonder if she is Hapa Aspie, as you call them. She is a wonderful grandmother, very loving and connects well with her friends, too. But she has always taken care of everything herself, even when Dad was alive. It's as if she doesn't realize we care enough about her to help out.

Without interrupting Helen's train of thought, I nod for her to continue.

I didn't really know Mom's parents since they passed away when I was very young, but I always thought one of Mom's brothers was very odd. You know what I mean? For example, only one of her brothers ever married. I always thought Uncle Adam was fun. He took us hiking and water skiing, and made the best buttermilk pancakes when I'd spend the night at his house.

But Mom's other brother, Uncle Bradley, was quite eccentric. He never married. He lived in a little travel trailer that he moved from town to town to follow his work. Now that I think about it, he was a mechanic, so why would he need to move all of the time? Unless he just preferred to keep his distance. Uncle Bradley always seemed happy to see us when he came to visit, which was about once or twice a year. It was never a holiday. He would just show up. He smelled like leather and wore cowboy boots and western shirts when no one else in the family did. Odd. I always thought of Uncle Bradley as kind and unassuming, but I never really missed him when he died. I don't think anyone did. That's why it was such a big surprise when Uncle Adam and Mom cleaned out his trailer.

Helen's voice trails off and she looks a little confused and sad. "What was the surprise Helen?" I ask. Helen continues.

Uncle Bradley didn't have any possessions that were worth anything except for his car. As a mechanic, he kept it in tip-top shape. Plus it was a classic car, you know—a two-toned 1955 Chevy. It was beautiful in yellow and white and not a scratch on it. I guess his car was his baby.

Helen seems to be wandering off a bit, so I nudge her back on topic. "Yes nice car I bet, but what was the surprise Helen? What surprised you when Uncle Adam and Mom cleaned out Uncle Bradley's trailer?" Helen looks at me with a new understanding surfacing.

Well Dr. Marshack, the surprise was that Uncle Bradley had pictures of me as a baby and little girl. He didn't have pictures of anyone else. He just had pictures of me that he put in little silver frames. Mom said he must have secretly stolen the pictures from her, because they were missing from her albums. If she had known he'd wanted those photos, she surely would have given him some, but he'd never asked. I remember him telling me how much he loved the color of my hair because it was exactly the same shade as his mother's, who'd passed away when he was a teenager. He made me feel special when he said that, and he'd said it each and every time he'd visited. In fact, I don't really remember him talking to me about anything else. So Dr. Marshack I suspect that my Uncle Bradley loved me very much, but I never knew it. Or perhaps he just loved my hair. So what do you think, could there be at least one Aspie in my family tree?

"You know Helen," I say, "Your intuitions are usually so accurate that I have to say you are probably right about Uncle Bradley. Of course he was never formally diagnosed and there's a lot we don't know about him. But it appears that he had some of the symptoms of Asperger Syndrome, such as trouble navigating the social world, or expressing love for his niece, or having an attachment to the color of your hair rather than to you. The lack of connection that you feel about your uncle is very telling. If he loved you enough to steal baby photos from your mother, and yet never told you he loved you, you are left with that typical empty and confusing feeling about the AS/NT relationship: You feel as if it isn't real at all. Maybe your mother is Hapa Aspie. You should talk to her more about this." Helen nods her approval.

It is not the least surprising that Helen may have grown up with Aspies (or a Hapa Aspie) in her family and then married a man with Asperger Syndrome. Grant's style may have been vaguely familiar to Helen. On the other hand how strange to choose a mate, because he reminds you of the parent you couldn't connect with. Some psychologists would take this a step further and say that Hapa Aspies choose an Asperger mate because of unresolved problems with their Aspie parent. In other words, Hapa Aspies continue to search for the connection they never had with their AS parent. Of course it is futile to seek that connection from another Aspie. As we have seen with Helen, this pattern only leads to disappointment, anger and even outright hostility toward the Asperger mate. Then the cycle is repeated with the children. Sad. Very sad.

Lessons learned

1. Hapa Aspies are children of AS/NT co-parents.

2. Hapa Aspies are stuck between worlds. Untreated by a trained psychologist, they live a lonely life of not fitting in as NTs or as Aspies. They can't seem to allow their authentic self to shine.

3. Aspie parents put their NT children in an emotional bind when they can't relate to the child's developing theory of mind, that we all have our own point of view—and that this point of view defines us.

4. NT children need their own psychologist from a young age and over a long period of time. This provides them with a neutral person who models a healthy relationship and teaches skills necessary to navigate the world of AS/NT relationships. A loving NT parent is not enough for the struggles a Hapa Aspie child has to go through.

5. The conflicts between Aspie and NT parents place the NT child in a no-win situation. The child needs a neutral party to help him or her find a way to BE genuine and still maintain a relationship with each parent.

6. By age 6, NTs are developing a theory of mind, but they are not mature enough to handle the disappointing disconnects with their Aspie parent. As a result, they blame themselves for their Aspie parent's inability to connect; hence at 6 years old, the child of an Aspie should be in psychotherapy to keep the boundaries clear.

7. Hapa Aspies often continue the search for a way to connect with their unavailable Asperger parent by marrying an Aspie, thus starting the Hapa Aspie cycle all over again.

CHAPTER EIGHT

Bullied or Bully?

Many parents of Asperger Syndrome children grieve over the bullying their child receives at the hands of other children. Many AS adults tell me that it took them decades to heal from this abuse and develop a modicum of self-respect. Think about the child who is a daily target on the playground, taunted by the other children, because of his smudged glasses or odd gait. Or think of the young AS girl who is hit in the head with a ball aimed specifically at her by insensitive classmates. Children can be cruel. But there is another side to the bullying that is often overlooked unless you are well versed in the dialectic of an Asperger Syndrome/neurotypical (AS/NT) family.

Those with AS engage in bullying, too; however, it is often directed only at those in their home. When NT adults or children complain about the abuse in their AS/NT home, they are often not believed. Until there is a grasp on the theories that explain: empathy disorders; the symptoms of mind blindness and *context blindness*; and zero degrees of empathy, it is very difficult for outsiders to understand the chaos and abuse that Aspies are capable of inflicting. In this chapter I explain how the rules of engagement can be applied to help Aspies regulate their emotional outbursts.

Parenting is the art of people-making

Having grown up with an AS mother, I certainly know firsthand how brutal and confusing the behaviors of an AS parent can be. It wasn't just the humiliation of making me wear bowling shoes to school, or never being hugged, or rarely being called by name. (Mom always called me Daughter.) When she raged, it was blood curdling. I learned to walk on eggshells around my mother, because I never knew for sure what would set her off. If I didn't make the bed with perfect "hospital" corners, or if I used too much soap for the dishes, she might come unglued. Her reaction was far from the "normal" way that my friends were scolded. It wasn't scolding, but abuse, when Mom would scream at me, using the foulest language, swear at me and accuse me of deliberately causing her harm. When I would make a normal childhood error, Mom would lay into me and accuse me of having made the mistake on purpose: "Just to spite me," she'd scream. I can still hear those words echoing in my ears. I'd been hurt that I had upset my mother, and I'd been hurt that she believed me to be so evil. It wasn't until decades later, with a contemporary understanding of Asperger Syndrome, that I realized my mother's limitations.

It's hard to hold up under that kind of verbal abuse. The belittling that AS parents indulge in is hard enough to take if you are an adult: A child feels gutted when their AS parent screams at her. Over and over again, NT parents tell me that their AS partners treat the children as if they have the psychological resources of an adult. Parenting is the art of *people-making*. Children are adults-in-training, and they need a little leeway to err. They don't have adult coping skills even if they are intellectually precocious. When a child makes a mistake, even a deliberate or manipulative mistake, the parent(s) should take this as a teaching moment not a hostile attack on their authority. The child may need a time out for misbehaving, but even then the parent has to look at the big picture. The big picture is that parents are intended to be mentors and guides and tutors for their children. Take this responsibility seriously.

The right way, the wrong way, and Dad's way

Helen is slowly coming to terms with the abuse she and her children endure as Grant's anxieties and obsessions rule the daily activities of the household. Here is one small example that demonstrates why life with an Aspie co-parent can be so tiring. Helen explains.

I can't really understand why Grant does things the way he does them. He is so inefficient. Take garbage day for example. He has these odd requirements, such as the cardboard has to be cut and folded only one way. Or all of the recycling and garbage have to be rinsed, sorted, stacked, and bagged in the kitchen before he takes it to the garage. And he counts all of the bags, too! This wouldn't be so bad, but it takes two days for Grant to gather up the household garbage and recycling!

Helen notices my eyes widen in surprise, then goes on.

Yes that's right. Grant tells me it takes two whole days to complete the recycling, because the kids and I are so wasteful and disorganized. So that means that the recycling sits in the kitchen for two days as Grant

fusses over it. We have to walk around it. We can't take it to the garage or Grant will holler. Even so, when he is tending the recycling piles, he is complaining loudly about us. He whines that he is not appreciated for how hard he works on this project. He says that if we would only cut up boxes—the right way—and place them in the required location—each day that we have a box—his life would be better. He seems angry that we have garbage at all, like he never contributes to it!

Oh it is true that I don't help much. When we do get a box, I just open the garage door and toss it out by the recycling bins. I do mean to get to it later when I have a moment, but Grant beats me to it—a full two days before garbage day!

Helen is well aware how ludicrous this situation is as she smiles and winks at me.

When Grant complains that we don't help him, I suggest that the twins are plenty old enough to help him gather up the garbage. For example, both Jason and Jasmine have started doing their own laundry— under my supervision of course, but they are getting the hang of it. But you know, I feel guilty putting the twins through their father's obsessive protocol for garbage. Nevertheless, I try to help Grant understand that the twins may organize the garbage a little differently than he would do it—maybe with the cardboard stacked under the glass instead of leaning against the garbage can—but that they can help and learn an adult responsibility. But that's not how it works with Grant. He doesn't really parent the kids; he orders them like little soldiers. They either do it his way, or they are screamed at and belittled beyond belief.

Helen's story reminds me of my mother, and my mind drifts a moment. All through my childhood, mother would joke about how stubborn was her father, Philip. She'd said they had an expression in their family: "There's the right way, the wrong way, then there's Philip's way." Mother had said that she and her brothers knew they had better do it Philip's way, or there would be hell to pay! In those days, that meant a "whoopin' " out behind the woodshed. I remember, as a child, wondering why my mother would laugh at her father over this rigidity when she herself operated under the same rules. Now I realize that this is an Asperger trait. *Context blindness* permeates almost every aspect of all relationships with Aspies. My mother hadn't been able to see how she was just like her own father, who was probably an Aspie, too. She definitely hadn't been able to see how her tirades about doing things the "right way" tormented me as much as she'd been tormented by her father.

Helen finishes her story.

Oh my goodness! Here's another example of how obsessed Grant is with the garbage. One time Jason was doing a pretty good job of staying out of Grant's way and still trying to help. One of Grant's rituals the night before garbage day is that he opens the door from the kitchen to the garage, preparing his route to the garbage and recycling bins. Jason dutifully lined up all of the household wastebaskets by the open kitchen door and started bagging them the way Dad had asked. Only he made one terrible error. Oh no!

Helen was mocking her husband as she continues her story.

'What are you doing?' Grant snarled at Jason. Jason had grabbed some of the plastic zip ties that came with the box of garbage bags and was sealing each bag neatly with one of them. 'Stop right now! How many times have I told you that we never use those flimsy zip ties. The garbage will just spill out when you lift the bag.' Grant was sweating profusely by this point. He gets so intense about this stupid little project that he puts all of his energy into it. It's nothing, but he makes it into the most important chore in the house. In fact he makes it so important that he can't possibly help me with anything else.

Jason looked flustered and worried that he was about to get a tongue lashing. He actually wanted to help out. You could see he was trying to enjoy a moment with his Dad, but Grant had to spoil it. I wanted to rescue Jason, but I have learned to stay out of things that could turn ugly if I interfere. Then, pointing to the open door into the garage, Grant orders, 'Get me the needle-nose pliers and those metal twist ties on the work bench over there.' Jason looked around but couldn't see the pliers or the ties. 'What are you waiting for Jason? What's wrong with you? Are you an idiot?' Grant gesticulated wildly with his left arm, pointing a finger in the direction of the workbench. 'Stop looking stupid. You couldn't find your head if it weren't screwed on!' Then Grant angrily marched over to the workbench, opened a drawer and found the needle-nose pliers. The twist ties were in a little plastic bin in the next drawer. Grant saves metal twist ties, even used ones. He doesn't believe in wasting anything. I suppose that is why he is so obsessed about the garbage. He hates waste.

Helen chuckles with the irony since Grant wastes so much time on the household "waste. I start to move in my chair and take in a breath as if to speak when Helen continues.

154

But wait. It's not over. Not only is Grant behaving like a madman over the garbage, acting so put-upon that he has to do this simple household chore and belittling his son for trying to help. He gets even deeper into his obsession with Jason. He hands Jason the metal twist ties; but before Jason can twist one around a bag of garbage, Grant howls again. 'No! Stop right there. Haven't I told you before? It's obvious. You can't seal the bags tightly enough if you don't use the pliers to twist the tie with precision.' Honest to God, he said that! 'Twist the tie with precision.' Can you believe it?

I learned long ago that I can't interrupt one of Helen's stories. She needs to wind it out to the end, so that for once she feels "heard" when she describes the AS eccentricities she lives with every day.

Helen slumps back in her chair. She lets her arms flop onto the armrests. She looks satisfied, gathering from the look on my face that she has adequately conveyed one more crazy-making experience with an Aspie co-parent. She sits up a bit and leans toward me and says:

It would be laughable, wouldn't it, if Jason weren't skewered by his father? That's the part that is the worst. Jason keeps getting the message that his father thinks he's incompetent. He's too young to truly understand that it is his father's problem. Jason 'gets it' that Jasmine has social problems, and he tries to cut her some slack. But he expects his dad to be—well, a dad. Grant rarely comes through. Over and over again, Grant obsesses with little details that send his anxiety through the roof. Then we all pay the price.

Later after the garbage detail was secured—like in the Army—I'd gone to Jason's room to console him. He said he was okay, but when I touched his shoulders, they were tight. I gently massaged his back and neck and shoulders to help ease out the tension. 'Jason,' I said, 'You are a great kid, and I am proud of you. Dad can be a handful. Don't let his obsession with the garbage unnerve you. I love you sweetie.' At that point I felt Jason's muscles give way, and he took in a deep breath and let it out again. You know that's how we all operate around Grant. We hold our breath and tense up our shoulders and back—until we can get away and finally exhale. This is no way to live.

If it feels like abuse, is it abuse?

Not many people can comprehend the mind-numbing abuse of living with an Aspie co-parent—unless they've lived it. Just as Helen described, one result of abuse, no matter what form the abuse takes, is waiting for the moment when you can exhale in safety.

Robin and Aldo's story is more about chronic neglect and rejection than about verbal abuse. Robin, the NT, feels the need to flee from the oppression—to be free. Oppression is indeed another type of abuse. If it feels like abuse, it might just be abuse.

Leaving an AS/NT marriage is especially hard for a parent when there are still minor children in the home. It's equally difficult when you know there will be absolutely no resolution. For NTs, who crave a win-win solution, divorcing an Aspie is excruciating, especially because Aspies so often believe there is the right way, the wrong way and "their way."

Robin has been divorced from her AS husband for nearly 10 years. In spite of the length of time that has passed and in spite of the fact that Robin asked for the divorce, she still has unresolved feelings about the marriage: This is not unusual for people in AS/NT relationships. Robin loved Aldo with all of her heart for nearly 15 years. She hadn't really wanted the divorce. But she had wanted her freedom. The oppression of a marriage without affection grew too unbearable. She'd half hoped that Aldo would change miraculously when she handed him the divorce papers.

Robin had told Aldo that she wanted a divorce several months before she filed. It had been on a Sunday evening, a time when, as was the pattern, they were off in their separate rooms while the children watched their last hour of TV before bed. Robin had gone to Aldo's room to talk, away from the children, so they wouldn't hear the discussion. Aldo had been shocked, of course, to hear that his wife wanted a divorce, because he had no idea there was a problem. He'd cried when she told him, and it had made Robin's resolve melt. When he'd asked her if she would go away with him for the weekend to a favorite mountain resort—just the two of them—to talk and work things out, she'd relented. She still loved Aldo, even if he was difficult to live with. If there was a chance to work things out, and keep her family intact, she was all for it.

As the week wore on, Robin heard nothing from Aldo about the weekend trip. He didn't talk to her about the divorce—or potential divorce. He didn't mention that he loved her either. For a man who had just been devastated by the divorce discussion, he was awfully calm. Out of mind, out of sight is the phrase that comes to mind at times like these. Aldo seemed to be content in his own little world of TV, computer, working, eating and sleeping. On Friday morning Robin and Aldo had the following conversation.

Robin had initiated the conversation of course. "Aldo I was wondering about our plans for the weekend. You haven't mentioned anything, so I wasn't sure what's up. What plans did you make? You know, are we going right after work tonight or leaving in the morning? Are we staying one night or two? What do you think I should pack? Should I pack mostly hiking clothes and maybe something dressy for one night out? You know, I just want to be ready. And what about the kids? I think they can stay with friends, but did you arrange anything?" Robin had left the planning to Aldo since he had made the invitation. Robin had hoped that Aldo's love for her would be motivation enough to plan their reconciliation weekend.

Aldo's response had been very casual for a situation where his marriage was at stake. "Oh that," he'd said rather nonchalantly. "Well I called the resort a couple of days ago, but they were all booked." Then he'd gone to the family room to watch TV.

Robin had been crushed. Did their relationship mean so little to Aldo that he couldn't even search for another lodge for the weekend? Was he really that helpless? It was then and there that Robin had decided to get the divorce and not be lulled back into believing that Aldo could change. She wanted her freedom, and she wanted her children to know that what she and Aldo had was not love.

It was three months before Robin could afford the divorce lawyer's retainer and deliver the papers to Aldo. He was, once again, in the family room with a beer, sitting in front of the computer and watching TV simultaneously. Robin had quietly walked up to Aldo, announcing his name as she'd approached so as not to startle him, "Aldo, do you have a moment?" One thing she'd learned long ago was never to approach Aldo abruptly. Aspies have exaggerated startle responses that can send them into a barrage of angry epithets. Robin hadn't wanted anger that night. She'd wanted both of them to remain calm.

"Sure Robbie. What do you want?" Aldo said cheerfully. He'd looked happy to see her, as if everything was the same as always—just the way Aldo wants it: Another example of out of mind, out of sight.

Robin was devoid of feeling at that moment. She was a woman on a mission. In her heart, she had cut the emotional ties to Aldo. Now she needed to handle the business end of things. She went straight to the point. "Aldo, I want a divorce. I have a lawyer." She paused to see if Aldo was listening. He sat there quietly, and the smile faded. "I filed

> Individuals with AS often close their eyes in order to think, but not just for a second like NTs. Aspies can remain with their eyes closed, saying not a word for minutes—while their NT partners are required to wait patiently for a verbal response.

the papers. Now we have to make plans to separate." Again Robin looked for signs of comprehension. Aldo gave no hint of a reaction just a steady look.

"Oh and the lawyer would like to know if you want to be served at work or if you would like to pick up the papers at his office? Or if you have your own lawyer, I guess the papers can be sent there."

Finished, Robin waited patiently for Aldo to make his move. Aldo seemed to be preparing something to say, because he didn't respond right away. He closed his eyes for a moment, and when he reopened them he said with a touch of surprise in his voice, "But I thought we were getting along better!" Then he fell speechless again. Robin had seen this behavior many, many times. Individuals with AS often close their eyes in order to think, but not just for a second like NTs. Aspies can remain with their eyes closed, saying not a word for minutes—while their NT partners are required to wait patiently for a verbal response.

Robin surprised herself with her quick comeback to Aldo's comment. It must have been the calm detachment that enabled her to be so patient with Aldo when he was making such immature statements. "I can see why you thought we were getting along better Aldo. I decided three months ago to stop talking with you. We haven't argued. We haven't made any mutual decisions. We haven't sat down in the evening and discussed our work days. There's been no conversation whatsoever. So I suppose that makes it seem to you like we are getting along better."

Aldo looked at Robin for a moment more and closed his eyes again as he pondered her analysis. Opening his eyes slowly and nodding his head ever so slightly in agreement, he said, "Now that you mention it, I think you're right about that. I don't remember us talking much lately." There it is again, a calm reporting of facts with no hint as to how Aldo is feeling. Nor does he express any empathy for his wife.

Bullying comes in many forms. When the Aspie lacks empathy and cannot fathom the mind of their loved one(s)—when they can only see the world from their own perspective—they are unable to rearrange the pieces of context surrounding their relationships to create a win-win solution. Helen described the controlling, verbally aggressive abuse that Grant leveled at Jason without any awareness of how this made Jason feel. Robin lived for years with neglect that felt like rejection. It beat her down emotionally. Aldo didn't realize he was neglecting his wife. He didn't realize that she and the children could not tell he loved them. How could they when Aldo spent night after night in front of the TV and his computer, never talking, never inquiring about their day, never curious about their feelings. The pain and sadness of it all still hangs in the air around Robin 10 years later. The oppression of abuse and neglect leaves an indelible mark on the soul.

There's a fine line between the bullies and the bullied

It may seem harsh to discuss the ways Aspies abuse and oppress their families, considering: the number of ASD children who are maliciously targeted every day at school; or the number of ASD young adults who struggle for independence, because of low self-esteem and social anxieties. But it is important to see the dialectic here. Theories about the cycle of abuse explain that there is a fine line between bullies and the bullied. Not all ASD children are targets of abuse for no reason. A *context blind* Aspie child may not read the social cues properly; hence may make the most disastrous decisions.

Max, for example, got expelled from summer day camp for assault-
ing another 10 year old. Max has Asperger Syndrome. He's a geeky
little kid with smudged glasses and a definite smell of feces about him.
Max has encopresis, an unfortunate disorder that is very common
among children with Asperger Syndrome. It is a condition that makes
bowel movements difficult. Researchers aren't entirely clear about the
etiology. It could be due to a virus, or food sensitivities or anxiety.
Because Max has problems with his bowels, he sometimes defecates in
his pants, unable to get to the bathroom in time. Sometimes he just
holds it in for days, so that he won't "forget" to go to the bathroom, or
have an accident. At these times his health is critically at risk.

With problems like these, it is no wonder that Max is ridiculed at
school and at day camp. Max was taunted for days at camp. One kid in
particular was quite the bully, and Max was not his only target. Over
and over again Max was called names such as, "tard" and "emo" and
"fart face," excluded from play with the other children, and generally
treated like a pariah. "Counselors" looked on, but they were young college students, who couldn't protect Max all of the time.

One day Max lost it. The bully pushed him one too many times,
and Max fought back. He kicked the other kid, clawed at him with his
finger nails and bit him on the arm before the counselors could pull
the boys away from each other. Both boys were expelled from day
camp for the rest of the week. The camp program had an obligation to
protect all of the children. Plus this was not a therapeutic camp but an
ordinary parks department program where certain behaviors could not
be tolerated regardless of a child's disability.

So how do you parent a child with AS regarding bullying? How do
you design the rules of engagement tightly enough to manage a tough
situation, such as bullying? How do you teach protection from abus-
ers? How do you teach other children to be respectful of individual

differences? How do you teach an Aspie child to manage his or her flood of emotions? This is certainly a conundrum.

The camp staff learned after the fight that Max's father had given him permission to fight back physically if he was bulled. I am sure that the father meant well, but does Max have the judgment to determine when and how to fight back? Obviously Max's father was not very specific about how to: fight back; stand up for oneself; and make a statement of strength in order to prevent future bullying. Consider how Max chose to protect himself. He waited until the abuse mounted to such a terrible level that he exploded. Then, instead of a typical boy scuffle, he attacked the other boy like a preschooler might. He scratched and bit him. Instead of teaching the other boy that he was a kid to be reckoned with, Max only humiliated himself further among his peer group with this immature behavior. No self respecting 10-year-old boy fights back by biting like a "baby."

Max's behavior reminds me of stories Helen has told about Grant. He has kicked the children and blamed it on them, saying things such as, "Jason started it!" He has threatened the children with comments such as, "I'll beat you with a big stick," or "I'll kick your face in." When Helen confronts Grant about this verbal abuse, he denies it is abusive. He claims the children know he doesn't mean it. But do they? Why does Grant believe that parenting is a series of verbal threats to do physical harm? The immaturity that Grant and Max demonstrate comes from Asperger Syndrome's *context blindness*; that is, the total inability to comprehend the nuances in social relationships. Plus it comes from years of living with an overactive nervous system that floods with fear when taunted by another human being.

The dark side of the AS child

Helen started her story with an explosion of tense emotion as she described her son, Jason's, alarm about what his AS sister Jasmine had done.

'Mom, Mom,' cried Jason. 'Jasmine just threw Ruthie down the stairs.' Ruthie is our dear little calico cat. Jason was so upset and needed me to take immediate action to protect the cat from his sister. I got up from my desk, hugged Jason's arm to give him some reassurance, then walked quickly toward Jasmine's room.

The cat was nowhere to be found, but I did find Jasmine, cool as a cucumber, sitting in her room listening to her iPod. I was direct. 'Jasmine,' I said. 'Did you throw Ruthie down the stairs?'

Jasmine turned slowly in my direction, pulled the earphones from her ears and looked at me as if to ask me what I was talking about. So I repeated myself, 'Jasmine, did you throw Ruthie down the stairs?'

'No,' she lied and put the earphones back into her ears. Jason was standing right next to me and couldn't believe it.

'She's lying!' he said. He was starting to cry. 'She's lying! I saw her. I heard Ruthie cry and howl when she hit the floor with a thud. Then she ran off somewhere and is hiding. I am worried about her. We have to find her and make sure she is okay.' Jason looked at me imploringly, 'Mom?' He wanted to be sure I believed him, because he was frightened for our cat. Again I reassured him with a gentle hug to his arm. Then we left to search for Ruthie.

I never did get a straight story from Jasmine, but I knew that Jason was telling the truth. The cat finally came out of hiding a little later. Ruthie seemed okay and snuggled up into Jason's lap for comfort. Dr. Marshack I am just horrified that Jasmine would do this. I know she has done it before. She has knocked the cat off her bed, and the poor thing nearly flew across the room. On another day when my car hit a bird, I felt just awful; then Jasmine quipped, 'Oh well, there are lots of birds.' How can Jasmine be so sensitive to her own needs, cry and have meltdowns at the drop of a hat, and yet be so callous and abusive at other times?

There's more to the Ruthie story, too. Jasmine got even with Jason for tattling on her. She took a pan of frosted cupcakes I had made for a school event and dumped them into Jason's new soccer bag. It was a lot of work to clean up that mess, but the worst was Jason's distress that his sister would be so vindictive. I do understand that Jasmine is high strung and easily distressed. I can imagine her overreacting to Ruthie if the cat caught her skin with a claw. But to deliberately plot to get even with her brother, that takes it to a new level of bullying.

Sometimes I think that Jasmine is abusive because of how Grant treats her, but you would think she would abhor abuse, not embrace it. And then there's Jason. Oh yes, he can get angry and quarrel with his sister, but he is not abusive. He's not a bully. Grant is just as harsh with Jason as he is with Jasmine, so I know that Jasmine's abusiveness just comes from within her—just like it does Grant. Am I on the right track here Dr. Marshack? And how on earth can I stop this runaway train? I am so worried for both of my children. I don't want either one to be a bully or a victim.

Helen sounds fatigued. The usual parenting approaches don't work in these situations. Helen gets very little support from Grant, so she's on her own to handle a complex parenting dilemma. If she went to him with this problem, Grant would just get angry with Jasmine and not recognize that he engages in the same type of abuse and bullying as his daughter. If Grant is angry with the kids or the cat he lashes out either verbally or with a physical assault. He has been known to backhand a child in front of others in a public restaurant. Similarly Jasmine became annoyed with the cat for some reason and threw it down the stairs. I have had more than one NT parent tell me similar stories. The AS child's anxiety escalates, and he or she becomes abusive and even retaliatory. With poor emotional regulation skills and low empathy skills, the AS child takes out his or her frustration on an animal or a sibling or a classmate.

Once again we see that when all of the attention is on the acting-out AS child or parent, the NT child is often left to deal with his or her grief over the abuse—alone. It is bad enough that Jason is worried about his pet, but he is also bewildered that his sister could be so cruel and vengeful. He loves his sister, too. Then what is he to make of Mom? Helen rescues Jason and the cat, but nothing really changes with Jasmine, or with Grant for that matter. The bullying continues. Mother and son hunker down together, perpetuating survivor mode.

Go beyond survivor mode

Getting beyond survivor mode and developing a parenting strategy to deal with bullies and bullying requires such a lot of work in an AS/NT marriage. It's not just about dealing with bullying from the outside world: NT parents are overwhelmed and fatigued by the bullying they and their children receive from AS family members. The NTs often are sandwiched between their Aspie partner and an Aspie child and/or an NT child. The AS partner and AS child are also caught in the crosshairs of societal expectations, peer pressure and their own overactive sympathetic nervous systems. It's no surprise that everyone in the family feels bullied.

Things can be done to stop the cycle of abuse and bullying, but you must be brave. You absolutely must establish firm rules of engagement for avoiding and handling abuse.

First, never tolerate abuse of any kind. Easier said than done, but there are few parents, Aspies or NTs, who would disagree with this basic rule. This is literally the most important rule of engagement regarding managing abuse. If voices are raised in anger, if a family member strikes another, if a pet is abused, if a family member seeks retribution—these are all violations of the basic rule of respectful and loving conduct. Be brave. Put aside your fear of the abuser and take a stand against oppression. Make a safety plan that includes removing yourself, your child, your pet or the abuser from the situation the minute abuse occurs.

Second, Aspies need to accept responsibility for their easily stimulated sensory systems. Being on the Autism Spectrum is not license to abuse. Medication and psychotherapy are requirements if those with AS are to manage their anxiety responsibly and not turn to bullying. They need to practice self-soothing behaviors, such as doing yoga breathing, taking breaks and timeouts, counting to 10, listening to quieting music and so forth. They need to ask for help when their emotions are gaining on them. And they need to apologize when they surprise and shock their NT family members. Being aware of their Asperger traits can help Aspies learn new skills to manage stressful moments quicker.

Third, I strongly recommend that Aspie parents turn over the lead role of parenting to their NT partner. Children are so unpredictable that the Aspie parent cannot keep up. With the many responsibilities of adult life, the Asperger parent gets easily overwhelmed and frustrated. They are not equipped to juggle the competing demands of working, getting household chores done, and teaching a child. When it comes to disciplining a willful child, the explosive adult Aspie temper is just too abusive. When I was a child, my NT father made that decision when my AS mother, in a moment of pique, had thrown a cast iron skillet at my sister's head. Then and there my father put his foot down: My mother agreed to refer all future child discipline to my father.

Fourth, this is not to say that the AS parent does no parenting whatsoever, but it should be circumscribed. The NT parent needs to handle those aspects of family life that require multi-tasking and spontaneous transitions, such as getting dinner on the table while breaking up a sibling quarrel. But the AS parent can be a marvelous softball coach or organizer of a Boy Scout camp out, because these events are planned ahead and very structured—something Aspies long for.

Fifth, AS parents need to be educated to offer as much verbal emotional support as possible to their NT partner. The details of all the NT spouse does to manage the household and keep things running smoothly are often lost on the AS spouse. My recommendation is to establish a rule about offering praise and delivering notes of appreciation daily.

Once again the antidote to bullying is to be brave and take a stand against oppression. If bullying has gone unchecked in your home for several years, you and your children have been living at a fever pitch of fear and survival for too long. You may have lost your inner strength. You may no longer believe in your ability to problem solve since nothing seems to work. Remember, solutions do not come from a place of fear. Fear just breeds more fear—and weakness. Instead of being fearful, seek answers where you can—where you are strong and smart and loving. For example draw confidence from your successes at work, or in your volunteer activities. Believe it or not you have healthy skills in these other areas that can be used at home with your family. You may be victimized, but you don't have to be a victim.

Lessons learned

1. Aspies and NTs alike can be bullies and can be bullied by Aspies and NTs.

2. Never tolerate bullying or abuse. Regardless of the motivation to bully, it is wrong and harmful to the child, to the marriage, and to the family.

3. If it feels like abuse it might just be abuse. Trust your instincts on this point.

4. Neglect is abuse, too. Over time neglect is a type of oppression that destroys love.

5. Seek psychotherapy for your family in order to conquer the bullying and to develop a successful parenting plan for a family of NTs and Aspies.

6. In fact, both the NTs and the Aspies need psychotherapy to learn methods for managing their distress, so that they don't decompensate into physical illness.

7. The bottom line is that NTs are better at quick transitions and parenting "on the fly" than are Aspie co-parents. Divide the parenting responsibilities accordingly.

8. Sadly, it is human nature to seek retribution when we feel wronged unless we are taught to hold to a higher moral code. Insist on teaching your children this moral code. Insist that your co-parent reinforce this code with his or her own behavior.

CHAPTER NINE

Are You Invisible?

One very striking result of growing up Hapa Aspie (Hapa Aspies are children of AS/NT co-parents.) is the development of a sense of psychological invisibility. I have heard many neurotypical (NT) partners complain of experiencing this phenomenon, too. What they mean by invisibility is that they feel ignored, unappreciated and unloved, because their *context blind* Aspie family member(s) is so poor at empathic reciprocity. As we have learned from Dialectical Psychology, we come to know ourselves in relation to others. This doesn't just apply to children. Throughout our lifespan, we continue to weave and re-weave the context of our lives, and our self-esteem, by the interactions we have with our friends, coworkers, neighbors and loved ones.

This is why it is so important for an NT parent/partner to get feedback from his or her spouse. A smile, a hug, a kind word, a note of encouragement—these are messages that reinforce the NT's self-esteem and contribute to a healthy reciprocity in the relationship. Without these daily reminders from their loved ones, NTs can develop some odd defense mechanisms. One is to become psychologically invisible to others and even to themselves. In this chapter, the NT spouse learns how to take back his or her life and to stop being invisible to others. With this knowledge, you may be able to help your NT children avoid becoming invisible.

Examples of invisibility

The following three vignettes provide an idea of what I mean by invisibility.

Rose Marie remembers one reason it wasn't so easy to invite friends over to her house after school. Her Asperger mother had the habit of locking the children out of the house for hours while she took her afternoon bath.

"My mother didn't seem to track time very well," says Rose Marie. "Even though she was home all day, she would just sit in her nightgown and read until the afternoon. When it would finally occur to her to take a bath, she would stop whatever she was doing and take one. It didn't matter if it was dinner time, or if I had a friend over to play. But if I did have a friend over to the house, my mother would make us go outside, then she would lock the door so that we couldn't get in to bother her."

I ask, "I am curious Rose Marie, would your mother let you stay in the house if you didn't have friends over? Did she somehow make a distinction about that?"

Rose Marie looks a little surprised that I understand something. "Well, yes she did," answers Rose Marie. "When there were no guests at the house, my mother was just fine taking a bath and wandering around the house naked. It wasn't that she needed so much time to take a leisurely bath, but that she liked to sit in her 'altogether' as she used to call it. She said she liked to dry off that way, and she really hated wearing clothes, too. So she would sit around 'drying off' for a couple of hours before she would reluctantly get dressed again. Sometimes I would find her sitting there at the kitchen table, naked and reading. Isn't that just strange Dr. Marshack?"

"Yes indeed Rose Marie," I say. "It is strange even though it is the kind of thing that Aspies do. They are often overly stimulated by bathing, or wetness, or the rubbing of certain textures of clothing against their skin. And the time thing—well, they just don't seem wired to be timely. They have difficulty coordinating timing with other things—like finishing her bath before you got home from school. But the most important thing to me about your story is how little Rose Marie must have felt. Did you feel invisible to your mother?"

Rose Marie's eyes widen as she makes a realization. "Yes that's exactly it, Dr. Marshack—invisible. Mom just had a way of ignoring whatever was going on except for her own perceptions. It wasn't that she didn't care about me. She just never got it that I felt abandoned a lot. Imagine how humiliating it was to bring a friend over to play and then get locked out of the house while Mom took a bath. Other mothers brought out cookies and milk for their kids' friends!"

Misty has another version of being invisible to her Asperger brother, Thom. Her big brother was an enigma to her all their growing-up years. He seldom paid much attention to her. She'd often wished he would even fight with her like other siblings, just so she could have some contact with him. But Thom was busy with motorcycles, stripping them down, rebuilding them, and winning the fascination of the other kids at school. Misty's father, loving that his son was so mechanical, had gotten Thom started working on dirt bikes and motorcycles at a young age. By high school, Thom had friends of a sort—lots of people who liked to hang out with him because of his mechanic skills.

One day Misty shared this brief anecdote about how her brother Thom literally treated her as if she was invisible. Thom carried a picture of Misty in his wallet. Occasionally he would pull it out and show it to his "friends." He kept that same picture for years, even into adulthood. Sounds nice doesn't it? Perhaps her Aspie brother loved her but just couldn't show it; however, the intriguing and sad part of this story is that the photo was not a picture of Misty at all. Thom had clipped the photo from a magazine and put it in his wallet. He'd told everyone it was his sister. When anyone had caught on that the photo was from a magazine, they'd asked, "Oh is your sister a model?" Thom had told them, "No," explaining that the person in the photo just looked a lot like his sister.

Then there's Zoe, and her father, Alan. Zoe, age 10, and her friend Kylee were playing a board game in the family room when Alan came into the room. The girls were sitting on the floor in front of the couch. Alan sat down at the computer, on the other side of the couch, apparently unaware that the girls were in the room. He turned on the TV with the remote control always conveniently located by his computer. He ran through a few channels to find something of interest. Then he turned to the computer and began work on a project.

Kylee started to say something to Alan to let him know the girls were in the room, but Zoe shushed her and grinned. She picked up the score pad from the game board and wrote Kylee a note, "See how long it takes my dad to notice we are here." Kylee gave her a conspiratorial smile and nodded agreement. For about 45 minutes the girls stifled giggles and wrote each other notes about what they were observing— all outside the awareness of Zoe's Aspie father.

They observed him laughing at something on the TV. They noted that "Dad scratched his butt." They listened to him sing to himself as he put paper in the printer. Alan left for a moment to get some food, but when he returned he was still unaware that the girls were watching him. They even peeked around the corner of the couch to watch him, and he was oblivious. The next time Alan went to the kitchen for a beer, the girls walked out of the family room and into the kitchen right behind him. Nonchalantly Zoe said, "So Dad watcha' doing?" Alan smiled at the girls, said hello to Kylee, and seemed totally unaware that anything was out of the ordinary.

Rose Marie, Misty and Zoe are invisible to their Aspie family members. It's not that their Aspies are trying to ignore them, but the Aspie *context blindness* makes tuning into the social environment next to impossible. Even worse, Aspies don't tune into the specific social cues that distinguish their loved ones from others. Rose Marie's mother knew that it would be inappropriate to be naked in front of someone other than her immediate family, but she was clueless how humiliated her daughter felt by being locked out of the house. Misty's brother may have observed that others kept photos in their wallets. Or perhaps he simply never removed the advertising photo that came with the wallet; however, Thom's lack of emotional attachment to the photo made his sister feel invisible to him. Zoe may have enjoyed pulling a prank on her father, but does she have respect for him? If something important comes up, and she really needs her father to be there for her, can she count on him? One wonders if she feels he is a fool, because when they are in the same room, she is invisible to him.

No one listens, because you are invisible

When I posted the topic of invisibility on my NT support group website for members to ponder and respond to, it was by far the hottest topic so far. (I'd started the online support group, Asperger Syndrome: Partners & Family of Adults on the Autism Spectrum, three years prior. To learn more about this group, visit http://www.meetup.com/Asperger-Syndrome-Partners-Family-of-Adults-with-ASD/.) Here is one woman's response:

> *Oh, this is an interesting topic. I have felt invisible for years–invisible to my husband. I talk, and he doesn't respond most times, and if he does, it's a grunt or one word or his favorite answer to questions [which is], 'I don't know.' I find myself repeating myself to see if he has heard me yet. What's bad is that I 'explain just a bit too much' to other people, probably boring them to death. I always have this feeling that they haven't heard me yet, so I keep talking. I knew something was wrong with that but didn't understand what was going on until I started reading the messages on this site.*

> . . . there is no "post-traumatic" to living with a *context blind* Aspie. The trauma of being invisible to your Aspie parent/partner occurs daily and is ongoing. For an NT, it's like being held an emotional hostage in his or her own home.

It is one thing to be treated as if you are invisible. It is another to come to believe it and act like it. In the field of trauma research, there are certainly a lot of explanations for the "psychic numbing" that results from suffering severe trauma. Until now, no one has really looked at the trauma suffered by NTs who are subjected to constant disregard by their Aspie family members. The result of this disregard is what I call, "invisibility." But what causes it? Is it a result of depression or post-traumatic stress disorder (PTSD)? The problem is that most depressions do not last years, and there is no "post-traumatic" to living with a *context blind* Aspie. The trauma of being invisible to your Aspie parent/partner occurs daily and is ongoing.

For an NT, it's like being held an emotional hostage in his or her own home.

In 1997, Families of Adults Affected by Asperger Syndrome (FAAAS) came up with the term, "Mirror Syndrome" and later "Cassandra Phenomenon" to explain the stress of living with AS family members. But these terms were still too vague. They did little to further the understanding of and support for NTs who were suffering. Currently, FAAAS favors the term, "Ongoing Traumatic Relationship Syndrome" (OTRS), which seems more specific to the lives of NTs partnering with Aspies. This definition definitely hit the mark with my group members when I presented it to them; however more research is needed to support the OTRS diagnosis. The FAAAS definition of OTRS from their website follows:

> "Ongoing Traumatic Relationship Syndrome (OTRS) is a new trauma-based syndrome, which may afflict individuals who undergo chronic, repetitive psychological trauma within the context of an intimate relationship."[34]

Within the context of the theories presented in this book, there is support for OTRS. If it is true that we come to know ourselves through the dialectic of our ongoing relationships, then the process of evolving a strong sense of self can be severely handicapped when the ones we love do not see us . . . touch us . . . listen to us . . . affirm us. Even if we come into a relationship with a strong sense of self-esteem, it can be demolished in short order by a partner or spouse who has an empathy disorder. If a grown person can develop traits of invisibility—like the woman who fell into the pattern of explaining too much—from living with an Aspie partner, think what happens to NT children or Hapa Aspies growing up with Aspie parents and Aspie siblings.

---

34   http://faaas.org/otrscp/

We learned in previous chapters about the importance of relating within the family in order for children to develop a strong sense of self-esteem. Rose Marie, Misty and Zoe experience being treated as if they are invisible on a daily basis. This experience sends some pretty conflicting messages about their self-worth and, in particular, their self-worth in relationships. If these children feel invisible to their AS parent, they can come to believe they deserve to be ignored.

In this chapter you will discover more stories of NTs who have Aspie parents and siblings. You'll see how invisibility haunts these NTs throughout their lives. You will learn methods for helping your NT children make adaptations and coping choices that are healthier. You will learn how to help them avoid believing that no one listens to them, because they are invisible.

Invisible slip and fall

Christmas lights twinkled in the lobby of the downtown Hilton Hotel. People were smiling and bustling around with the excitement of the season. Even though the evening darkness was falling outside, inside was warm and festive with red and green decorations and holiday music. I felt like singing the classic Christmas tune, "Silver Bells." You know, the tune about, "City sidewalks, busy sidewalks," or the part about, "Silver bells, silver bells, it's Christmastime in the city." I was in the heart of the city during the holiday season—when we all feel just a bit more hopeful about our future. We wish for true love, a warm and hearty Christmas dinner with family, resolution to problems, and so forth. And we kind of believe, like little children who believe Santa grants wishes, that our heartfelt wishes will come true. I felt that warm spirit as I crossed the lobby to the bar.

I had arranged to meet a friend for a drink in the Hilton Bar after a day of seminar at the City Convention Center next door. I'd arrived about 15 minutes early, enough time to "freshen up" in the ladies room. I'd walked into the bar, crossed the hardwood floor past the bartender and turned right to enter the hall to the restroom. I'd barely made the turn past the bar when I'd slipped. As I'd fallen, I'd thought to myself, "It's okay. Just relax. Take the fall nice and slow." And that is what I'd done. Both feet had slipped out from under me, the left one first, then the right. I'd leaned slightly to the right. As I'd hit the floor, I'd landed on my "bum" and hit my head on the wall to my right.

I sat on the floor for a few moments, gathering my wits and making a plan. I looked over my shoulder at the bartender, who just stood there with a blank look on his face. As if to answer his unspoken question, I said, "Yes, I fell." He didn't make a move to help me. No one in the bar got up or expressed any concern. They just stared incomprehensibly. So I pulled my knees up and under me, and with my right hand against the wall, I pushed-pulled myself up off the floor.

No one moved at all. No one spoke a word. I turned and walked toward the bartender and said, "I just fell. There must be something slippery on the floor there," as I pointed to the spot where I'd fallen. I hoped that he would acknowledge me—and the danger. He leaned past the bar a bit, looked over his shoulder in the direction of the floor and said in a monotone voice, "Oh yes. I can see a spot on the floor." Then he turned back to the bar and tended to his other customers.

Since I got no help or acknowledgement, I continued on to the ladies room. Upon returning to the bar, I found a table and waited patiently for my friend to arrive. I guess I am invisible. At least to the Hilton Bar patrons.

I never really thought about invisibility before I learned about my mother's Asperger Syndrome. I realize now that I have been invisible all my life, and I believe it is a condition that plagues a lot of NT people in Asperger/NT families. In *Going Over the Edge?* I describe an incident when Helen passes out on the bedroom floor but her husband doesn't even acknowledge her fall. When you live with people who do not acknowledge you, one way to cope is to become invisible—strong, independent, self-sufficient—yet unseen. Even though I am a busy professional with a full schedule, I frequently have experiences where others ignore my needs. It is as if I send out signals giving permission to ignore me. Otherwise, who in their right mind would ignore a 60-year-old woman who has just fallen in a Hilton Bar? Yet my story is true.

Now, I can attribute my invisibility to my Asperger mother. I share my sense of invisibility, because, in this book on parenting with a partner who has Asperger Syndrome, I think it is important to hear from those of us who grew up with an Aspie parent and/or an Aspie sibling(s). It is such a different world, hardly believable. My office manager, Michelle, has a darling way of describing some of my stories of invisibility. She says, "The reason people have such a hard time <u>believing</u> your stories is that they are <u>unbelievable</u>." So true. There is no better word for them than "unbelievable." I hope this book brings the phenomenon of invisibility into the light, so that those of us who were invisible children are finally heard and believed—and visible.

Three traits of invisibility

If you noticed, when I fell in the Hilton Bar, I had a plan of defense even as I fell to the floor and hit my head: Calm, cool and collected in the face of adversity. That's not bad if your goal is to be a Steven Seagal-type of unfeeling superhero. One thing I learned from being ignored and misinterpreted by my Aspie mother is how to handle a crisis. I am absolutely terrific in a crisis. That's because, as a child, if you don't think your parent will help you, you start to develop methods for taking care of yourself. As a result, I developed an interesting blend of three traits of invisibility.

- First, is what I call the Zen Master. I became invisible, so that I could avoid my mother's tirades. Please don't mistake this trait as some form of real Zen mastery, although it is certainly useful when you are behind enemy lines.

- Second, is what I call the Tough Cookie. I learned to toughen up since Mom didn't seem to notice that I needed anything. All of my life I have been called a Tough Cookie. This trait has a terrific warrior quality: People leave tough guys alone.

- Third, is what I call No Fear. My own feelings became invisible to me. This is similar to the psychic numbing quality reported by sufferers of PTSD. Having No Fear is another powerful trait for coping. My ex-husband used to say about me, "You walk where angels fear to tread."

But what about love and caring and creative self-expression? No room for that when you are invisible. While many children of Aspie parents are invisible—even to ourselves, there are rumblings of visibility going on beneath the surface. For example, when I turned 18, I became aware that I was very depressed. This is not uncommon for teenagers just about to launch into adult life. It can feel frightening to face the unknown. With supportive parents, teenagers make this transition in a healthy way. Healthy parents send their children the messages that: they believe in them; they will provide backup if anything goes wrong; they are loved and cherished no matter what mistakes might be made. But when a child has an AS parent who sends mixed signals, he or she can feel so totally abandoned and insecure that they don't know what to do. That was me.

When I was 18, I epitomized the Zen Master. I used to come home from school each day and engage in the following ritual. I filled a small dessert bowl with Cheezit crackers and took it to my bedroom. I put earplugs in my ears to dampen any sound. I just wanted to shut out reality altogether, because it was so painful to be alone. I wrapped myself in two blankets. The warmth and bulk was comforting—like Temple Grandin's hug machine.[35] Plus I always felt cold, and the blankets warmed me. Then I crawled into bed with my Cheezits and my homework and read. I think I came to dinner when my mother called me, but I really don't remember. I was obviously very depressed. After dinner I spent the rest of the evening in my bedroom, again with my earplugs and my studies—all the while huddled in blankets—being as invisible as I could get.

This went on for months. I was depressed, cold—and invisible to my AS mother. I was descending into oblivion. In the spring, something stirred in me, and I realized that I needed to stop this madness. I got an idea. Tired of being depressed and invisible, I decided to look for a job and be with people. I looked in the newspaper for job postings and applied at Newberry's, the kind of place we used to call a "dime store." They hired me on the spot. I loved it. I was a "floater," assigned to any department that needed a sales clerk. I worked in women's wear and at the candy counter, in jewelry and yard goods, you name it. I found myself looking forward to work and the friends I made there. Plus I felt smart for a change. I never understood why the other sales clerks couldn't figure out how to make change for

---

35   Temple Grandin is a noted autistic and author on the subject of autism spectrum disorders. Because of her sensitivity to human touch and yet her need to be embraced, she designed a machine that gently squeezes her body. You can learn more about Dr. Grandin at www.templegrandin.com

customers, or why they found it so hard to figure out how much candy a customer could buy for 56 cents. It didn't take long for the store management to recognize that I was a bright, personable young woman. Within three months, they promoted me to Night Manager! What better job for a Tough Cookie.

Wow! What a change from the depressed, invisible teenager who hid in her room, cold and all alone. I wish I could tell you that the job at Newberry's solved everything, but I can't. While this step helped me realize that there was more to me than my AS mother ever could understand, it took me decades to really resolve my cold and unloving childhood. Apparently the legacy of childhood invisibility lingers to this day, as evidenced by my Christmastime fall in the Hilton Bar.

A couple of years after the Cheezit spell, I had the opportunity to ask my mother what she thought about that time in my life. I'd wondered if she'd even noticed that I'd hidden away in my bedroom, shivering under two thick blankets. Had she suspected I was depressed? Why hadn't she reached out to me? Had she cared at all? Here's the conversation we had.

I'd asked, "Mom, remember when I was 18 and hid in my bedroom for months until I got the job at Newberry's? I was wondering what you thought about me at that time? You know, I just ate Cheezits after school and didn't see a soul. No friends, nothing. So what did you think was going on?"

Mom had given me that flat Aspie look as she'd thought through my question. She'd drawn a puff on her cigarette, blown out the smoke and finally responded in her typical monotone, "Well, you always were a quiet child." Then she'd picked up her magazine to begin reading again. Before turning completely away from me, she'd taken a puff off her cigarette again, and blown it in my face as if I wasn't there at all. The conversation was finished. I hadn't specifically asked for emotional support, so she'd given none—just offered her opinion as I had asked. Very Aspie. Very *context blind*. Is it any surprise that I adopted a style of being invisible?

That time, I'd been undaunted by her aloofness or the cigarette smoke. I had gained courage from my experience at Newberry's, and I was not going to let fear of my mother get in my way. I'd tried another approach. I'd ramped up the emotional quotient on the next question. "Mom, didn't you worry about me though? Did you think that maybe I needed a hug or some comfort? I mean I was depressed and going nowhere with my life!"

My mother had looked at me with that same faraway look I saw on the bartender's face at the Hilton. She'd listened, but she had no comprehension that feelings were involved. It hadn't registered with her that I'd been hurt then—and was hurting still. I'd taken a deep breath and waited for her response. "Well let's see," she'd said, closing her eyes to think for a moment, a very characteristic Aspie move. When she'd spoken again a few moments later, I'd realized she had analyzed my question and was offering a reasonable explanation. She'd said, "You were never a cuddly baby. I remember as a toddler you didn't like to sit on my lap. Whenever I picked you up, you squirmed to get away. So I just assumed you liked to be by yourself." I'd gotten another puff of smoke blown into my eyes.

Good analysis, Mom, but way off the mark. Every toddler squirms to get away, to test the boundaries of their independence. But they run right back and want to be held—for a moment—before they venture out to explore again. Parents are a toddler's safety zone. The child believes he or she can venture out only if they know that they can always run back to Mommy or Daddy for comfort and safety. Not so with an Aspie Mom, who takes everything literally and can't read her child's motivations or even understand normal child development. My mom had read all kinds of child and baby care books when I was little, but she'd been unable to put the pieces of context together within her own family. I guess she'd been reading about someone else's child in those books, so none of the advice had applied to me—or to her.

So there you have it. My mom never noticed my descent into depression, even though she was aware of an interesting pattern. Aspies have a marvelous ability to notice patterns even in human behavior. The problem is that they don't always recognize the emotional meaning to the pattern, and they rarely comment on the meaning.

The real question is: If a parent doesn't notice the emotional needs of his or her child, does the parent care? How can you really love your child if you don't engage with them in their emotional world? Can you love your child even if you don't relate and only notice concrete patterns? How does a child learn they are loved and lovable if they have a parent who doesn't demonstrate empathy? *True empathy* requires going beyond observing the pattern of human behavior. *True empathy* requires connecting all of the empathy circuits in the brain and responding appropriately to loved ones. *True empathy* means that out of the entire context of our lives, our loved ones (children and spouse) are front and center, not part of the background.

No explaining

I have heard many stories about the development of traits of invisibility from adults who grew up with an Aspie parent or who are co-parenting with an Aspie. They report being lonely at work and in their personal lives. Like Helen, these invisible NTs are often very accomplished people, but the cloak of invisibility they wear robs them of true intimacy. Carmen's invisible nature takes on a different appearance than mine. Carmen is a delightful, attractive, 37-year-old woman. She has a casual grace, an engaging smile, and a sense of humor that keeps you laughing throughout a conversation. She is definitely no wallflower, but she doesn't steal the show either. She has a way of making you feel special with her kind humor.

No one knows Carmen's pain. It is startling to realize that she has personal problems when she presents with such a cheerful demeanor. When Carmen first came to me for therapy, she wanted help with anxiety and Attention Deficit/Hyperactivity Disorder (ADHD). She hadn't seemed all that distressed to me. She'd been laid off of work, so that could have been contributing to her anxiety, but otherwise she was very psychologically resilient. I wondered what she really wanted and why she kept coming back to therapy. She was making good choices as far as I could tell, so why therapy? When Carmen began to tell me a bit about her childhood, I doubted her self-diagnosis of ADHD. Beneath the superficial ebullience was a woman who desperately wanted real love and connection.

So at one of our appointments, I asked about her childhood family. "You know Carmen, I have been puzzled about your situation and wondered if there are experiences in your childhood that may have contributed to the problems you want help with. Could you tell me . . . ? She begins:

Oh that is such an interesting question Dr. Marshack.

Carmen broke in before I was finished speaking and began her well-thought-out explanation.

Yes my childhood changed so much when our family moved from a small town to a larger one. I was only 6, and the move made such a big impact on me. I left all of my friends and felt so alone in the new town. I just never got over it. That explains why I don't really have friends today either.

Carmen smiles at me and nods affirmatively, very confident of her analysis of the situation. It seems rather superficial to me. I gently confront her. "Carmen, it seems a bit extreme for a child to be totally shut down for a lifetime, because of a move her parents made when she was 6. Yes I am sure that you were affected and felt a little lost at first. But certainly you could make the adjustment. You are so outgoing and friendly today. It just doesn't add up to me."

With a look of genuine concern for my confusion, Carmen ventures another analysis.

I know it seems strange, but it is the truth. My mother was always so self-absorbed that she never understood how much I counted on my old neighborhood friends to be there for me.

This time I interrupt. My conversations with Carmen are like that. Rapid fire exchanges of analysis—no feeling—then a little humor thrown in. "Wait a minute Carmen. What do you mean your mother was self-absorbed?" I'm getting suspicious that Carmen's mother was more than just a bit self-absorbed.

Oh yes. Everyone in the whole family jokes about Eloise. Gosh she would forget where she parked the car. One time she parked the car with the keys in the ignition and went shopping. Everyone has done that a time or two, but I betcha they didn't leave the parked car running! Oh the stories we tell about her when she is not around! I mean she was just so tuned out that she would forget to pick me up from choir practice, or forget to pack my lunch, or let me stay up late watching TV, because she was deep into reading a book. So you see it was just very difficult to leave my home town, because I'd counted on the neighborhood families to be like my extended family. It just wasn't the same in the new town.

I look at Carmen and try to get past the glibness. "Carmen, I wonder if your mother was more than just self-absorbed. Do you think she was just unaware of your needs? And where was your father when your mother forgot you at choir practice?" Carmen offers yet another explanation.

Well Dad has passed on now. He was a good man, but divorced Mom when I was about 10. He was alcoholic, so I think he left most of the child care to Mom. I liked my father's jokes though. He always made me laugh. But he never really helped me with anything. He was kind of old school that way and left the parenting to Mom.

Carmen conveys no real emotion, just a steady stream of explanations. "Carmen, I notice that you keep explaining everything but not really getting to your feelings about all of this. It sounds to me like you had a lonely childhood with an alcoholic absent father and a self-absorbed and indifferent mother. I don't think the move at age 6 was what turned you inward. I think what happened at age 6 is that you woke up and realized that your parents wouldn't be there for you. That is scary for a little girl. If she can't count on her parents to back her when she moves to a new town, how can she reach out to make new friends? She needs to know that her parents will keep her safe and love her no matter what happens in the new neighborhood and new school. But you didn't get that support did you?"

I notice tears welling up in Carmen's eyes. She looks at me in amazement and the ever-so-charming smile fades from her face. She whispers,

Oh Dr. Marshack, no one has ever understood this before. I was a lonely little girl, and I still am, and I can't figure out what to do about it.

Over the next few weeks, Carmen and I talk in depth, much more than we ever have. As she reads more about Asperger Syndrome, she comes to realize that the diagnosis fits her mother to a "T." We discuss how she has been affected by the verbal abuse from her Asperger mother and the intermittent emotional support from her depressed alcoholic father. Her sisters were no help to her. As the youngest in the family, she was bullied by the older siblings, who were trying to satisfy their own lonely feelings. With Mom absent due to her lack of empathy skills and Dad absent due to self-medicating with alcohol, Carmen had to fend for herself.

One of the ways Carmen found to protect herself was to use her considerable intelligence and sense of humor to gain at least a bit of positive attention. She can entertain people for hours with tales of her family, especially her mother's eccentricities. In therapy, Carmen creates the most elaborate explanations of why her life is the way it is. But none of this explaining creates the loving connection Carmen is searching for.

Among intelligent and well educated people, it is quite common to come to "understand" and then explain why your life has turned out the way it has. But these explanations change nothing. In fact these explanations tend to seal fate. Carmen found a way to be invisible to others by having a quick explanation for everything. All of her explanations formed a drape of invisibility; hence locking the door to new relationships. People come to know Carmen only through explanations about her past. No one has had the chance to know the woman she is today.

No complaining

One of my Aspie clients comes from the southern United States. His mother taught him an old fashioned southern euphemism that is oddly appropriate for NTs like Carmen: "No explaining; no complaining." If you think about it, this homespun advice makes a lot of sense. Explanations are used as a defense against the sadness of being ignored. Explaining and complaining are defensive maneuvers that we use when we feel trapped: They are attempts to prove to ourselves that we are okay; whereas if we are truly okay, then what is there to defend?

I have heard plenty of explaining and complaining from NTs with Aspie parents or partners, and it is usually the explaining that NTs cling to. Complaining is more a victim kind of thinking. Complainers accept that they are trapped, but they don't like it—and they tell everyone about it. Blaming others takes the burden of responsibility off the complainer; though it still makes them feel out of control of their lives. Analysis and explanation provide a sure-fire way to feel in charge of a situation. When an NT child takes responsibility for her parent's actions, it gives her a false hope that she can change the parent. It's not true of course, but it feels much better than complaining.

Carmen's therapy took a positive turn when I gave her this assign-ment. "Carmen, I want you to stop explaining or complaining. All you can talk about is now—what you are feeling or hearing or seeing or smelling. You can't analyze. You can't blame others or yourself. You can't judge either. No complaining. No explaining."

Carmen says, "This is a wonderful assignment. This is exactly what I need, because my, mother . . ."

Interrupting Carmen, I laugh gently and say, "There you go again explaining. Remember now, the minute you say, 'because,' you are probably launching into an explanation once again. Stop it. Take a deep breath. Begin again."

Carmen and other invisible NTs in AS/NT relationships really need this assignment. It enables them to experience feeling truly okay, ac-ceptable, fully alive—even without an explanation or a complaint. The no explaining, no complaining exercise helps with learning how to "just be." That opens to NTs another, "visible" world to live in. And what a wonderful world to offer our Hapa Aspie children—a world that holds the opportunity to know that they are loved whether or not they have a good explanation. Explanations are for the invisible. When you feel free to show the world who you really are, no explanations are necessary.

Lessons learned

1. When an Aspie parent cannot reciprocate a relation-ship or acknowledge a child's frame of mind, then the child can develop a strong sense of feeling unimport-ant or being invisible.

2. When the NT child does not just feel visible to their AS parent, they can come to believe they deserve to be ignored. In fact, they can send signals to others that they are invisible and should be ignored.

3. Forgive yourself even if you can't always stop being invisible. You learned this defensive trait a long time ago. The first step to reclaiming your life is to observe those behaviors that render you invisible.

4. The best description of what NTs are feeling in AS/NT families is Ongoing Traumatic Relationship Syndrome (OTRS).

5. You and your children should not be part of the back-ground in the life of your AS co-parent. You should be in the forefront.

6. Do what you can to honor your NT children. They need to know that you really "know" them—even if you are preoccupied with caring for your Aspie family member(s). Try to spend time with your NT children away from the Aspie family members. This will allow the NTs to relax and trust that their perceptions of reality are accurate.

7. The NT child, who has experienced feeling invisible to their Aspie parent, needs the support of a psychologist who can draw out the child's authentic self.

8. No Explaining. No complaining: You don't need these coping mechanisms. Your perceptions and intuitions are just fine. You may see things differently than your AS partner or parent, but neither of you is wrong. It's okay to foster differences and independence. Think differently. Be different. BE.

CHAPTER TEN

Can You Teach Love?

This question from Helen brings up the most important element in parenting—the art of loving your child, so they grow up confident and strong in their sense of self. What does Helen do when her daughter, Jasmine (a child with Asperger Syndrome), tells her mother that she isn't sure what love is? In this chapter you will learn that a basic human experience, such as giving and receiving love, is not so easy in Asperger Syndrome/neurotypical families.

Love is more than feeling it (emotional empathy). Love is more than talking about it (cognitive empathy). Love is more than systemizing a moral code to live by (as many Aspies do to compensate for their empathy disorder). Love is more than practicing the rules of engagement (although politeness helps). The answer to Helen's question is worth exploring in a real and deep and heartfelt way. In this chapter we move beyond the theories and science of empathy and social learning to see how Helen, Vivian and Todd, Anne Marie and Tony work through the dilemmas of teaching and experiencing love with their children and each other. This is the most profound work a parent can do.

How do you parent the cell phone generation?

Helen tells another story.

I overheard a couple of moms engaged in a light-hearted discussion when I walked over to where the parents sit for the game. You know, the parents have to sit on the other side of the field since the coaches have to maintain 'crowd control' with us unruly, disrespectful parents. So we aren't allowed to sit on the same side as the team and give the coach advice or run to rescue our little darlings when they get the stuffin' kicked out of 'em. Ha!

Helen has a delightful sense of humor when she isn't deep in her own lonely world. I was pleased that she could describe a joyful parenting time, such as sharing her child's soccer game with other enthusiastic parents. Helen really appreciates Jason's soccer training, because the coach is a family man, who makes sure the game is not just about winning. It's mostly about having fun. Jason has played with the same team for five years, so they really are like family. While Jason plays soccer, Helen can sit with the other parents, rain or shine, and enjoy the camaraderie of parenthood.

Helen continues her story.

So I unfolded my chair, put my purse under the seat, and laid my bell and pom-poms next to me on the grass while Jason ran across the field

to his teammates. Yes indeed, I am one of those crazed Soccer Moms: I love the game so much that even now I still ring the bell for a goal and shake my pom-poms. Jason, at age 15, always acts mortified when I do this stuff, but his friends love it. Sometimes his teammates call over to me from the 'bench' and say, 'Get ready to ring the bell Mrs. H!' It's their signal that they are confident of victory. Plus, I know that Jason is not too old for the bell and pom-poms, because he always asks me, nonchalantly, if I have everything before we leave for his games. And I know he doesn't mean just his cleats!

The game turned out to be fun, but there was this bit of sadness that came over me when I rolled up to these other moms. They were sharing amusing anecdotes about their daughters. One anecdote in particular made me grieve for the loss in my relationship with Jasmine. You see, this mom was laughing about her daughter's teenage rebellion. It is a very cute story, but sad for me.

'You won't believe what my Angela did yesterday!' said the first mom.

'No! Tell me,' said the second mom, looking on eagerly.

The first mom was laughing when she described what had happened. She said, 'Well I had to take the baby to the pediatrician, so I picked up Angela after school and headed out. Angela was bored, of course, so when we got to the doctor's office, she'd asked if she could play games on my cell phone. I'd said, 'Why not do your homework while you wait?' Of course I'd gotten one of those 'Oh- My- Gosh-Mom' looks and a heavy sigh. So I handed her my phone, checked in at the front desk and sat down to wait for our appointment.'

By then another mom had joined us and was listening and smiling, too, waiting for the story to get juicy. We were all leaning forward in our folding chairs in anticipation of the punch line. So the first mom says, 'After awhile I noticed that Angela was texting a friend without my permission. I scolded her but told her she could continue if she was responsible and stopped when I asked her to. We do have unlimited texting, *because it is kind of handy, but I don't want Angela to get addicted to texting. If she had her own phone it would be a nightmare!'*

Helen rolls her eyes as if to say, "You know how kids are. They have to text their friends day and night." I concur silently with a smile and a nod of my head because we all know what a phenomenon cell phones are, especially for children. "But what makes you sad about this day Helen? It sounds like you were having fun," I say.

Helen explains the amusing part.

Well here's the funny part. This young pre-teen was texting her friend alright, but she was complaining about her mom and using her mom's cell phone to do it! She texted things like, 'My Mom is such a retard,' and 'She won't let me have my own cell phone when everyone else has one!' But here's the clincher. When the mom asked for her phone back, the daughter made one last text that read, 'Mom wants her cell phone back. What a retard. She needs to see a doctor to get her brains fixed!' Only it was all texted in that weird teen-text shorthand.

Angela's mom had found the texts later in the evening when she'd had time to scroll through her phone to see what her daughter had been up to. She saved the texts and showed us. Oh my! We all burst out laughing. During little breaks in the soccer game, all of us would look at each other and laugh again. It was so funny I still chuckle when I think about it.

Even funnier was the part when she'd confronted her daughter. The kid had been stunned that she had been caught, as if her mother really did need to have her 'brains fixed.' Eventually, I guess the daughter made an embarrassed apology to her mom. Thank goodness, at least this child has some respect for her mom. Why do kids think their parents are stupid anyway? Oh I know that is the same question Socrates was asking in ancient Greece. Teens are teens no matter the century.

Is it love if they don't love you back?

Just as Helen ends this anecdote with a huge smile of amusement and another roll of her eyes, a flicker of sadness crosses her face. She restores her composure before the tears form. As she continues her story, I better understand the sadness.

Oh Dr. Marshack I only wish that I could scold Jasmine for using my cell phone to send her friends snarky remarks about me. But Jasmine doesn't have any friends at all. Not even one person to text like all of the other girls do. She lives in her room, with her computer and her music, but she will not reach out anymore to the other girls. When she was younger, I took her to play group, then Girl Scouts, and choir practice and music classes. We even tried soccer, but she begged me to take her out when she was frightened by all of the aggressiveness of the game. As she has grown and now is 15, she has dropped all of these activities, and the other girls have stopped calling, because she doesn't call back. When those other mothers were laughing at Angela's transgression, I wondered if they know how lucky they are.

You know it is not just that my heart is breaking because Jasmine is lonely, but it's about me, too. I can relate to Jason and he to me. He makes me laugh and looks to see the smile on my face, just to be sure we are connecting. Jasmine rarely does this. I was so overjoyed when I gave birth to Jasmine. I was looking forward to doing all of the girl things with her. I don't mean prissy or preppy stuff. I mean just sharing with each other the discovery of growing through the stages of girlhood. If she *wanted to play soccer and wear makeup and write computer programs, it doesn't matter if it is [or isn't] traditional girl stuff. It's the sharing and relating and connecting and bonding with her that I miss. I love her, and I know she loves me, but she doesn't love me back. Do you know what I mean?*

The grief is palpable. How on earth do you grieve the loss of the mother/child relationship when you still love your child? Once again I have a new appreciation for the loneliness and disconnect in Helen's world. She is learning to love Jasmine in a much different way than other mothers love their NT children. Loving a child with Asperger Syndrome means being an unconditionally loving caregiver. When your child is not wired for empathy, the love that may be in his or her heart is seldom given back in ways that make an NT feel loved.

Furthermore, how do you explain these things to other parents? Do you pretend, as Helen did, to understand? She'd nodded her head when the other Soccer Mom had told her story. She'd laughed at the mom's anecdotes. She'd rolled her eyes at the punch line. But Helen had had no cute anecdotes to share. It's not that Jasmine can't tell a joke or laugh with her mother: Once again we're reminded that the meaning of life is in the small stuff—like a daughter texting a girl friend.

Love takes many forms. One is the bond that develops over time between childhood friends who grow up together. Jasmine may never know that bond, because of her social anxiety. Likewise Helen was looking forward to a mother and daughter bond that would grow tighter over a lifetime—to the point when they would become adult friends. Even with its ups and downs, there is nothing stronger than a mother/daughter bond. When you can't share those small moments with your child, it is tragic.

Love is not an acquisition

Helen has more to say on this subject of love. She has a puzzled look on her face as she explains the unique way that her daughter thinks about love. "Dr. Marshack, Jasmine has told me more than once that she is not sure she knows what love is. I was surprised the first time she told me this, but I can sort of understand what she means. Now that I understand better how Asperger's works, I realize that her empathy disorder and *context blindness* get in the way of sharing her love with me, and even letting me love her back. I hope that she feels the love in her heart for me, her brother and her dad; because I show her all the time that I love her. But without having connecting cognitive and emotional empathy, how can Jasmine have reciprocity in relationships? How can Jasmine ever learn to love and know that she is loved? Dr. Marshack, can you teach love?"

This last question takes me by surprise. I don't think I had ever considered teaching love overtly, but Helen has a good point. You can drill in social skills, such as: setting the table properly; sending thank you notes; or formally addressing an adult. You can manage temper tantrums with simple behavior modification techniques (well maybe some of them). But love is something that we assume is natural. The NT mother feels love even before her child is born, but especially when she gazes into her newborn's eyes and the child gazes back. The first smile, the first "coo" from Baby are evidence of love coming back to the mother from the child she adores. It's no longer just about being fed and diapered. The baby is loving her back. And what father has not fallen head over heels in love with his child the first time he or she calls him "Da Da?" Even changing diapers becomes a labor of love to a father who thought he could never stand "poopy" diapers—all because his child loves him back.

Over the years children learn about all kinds of love, not just familial love. They love their friends because they are fun to be with, and they share the excitement of childhood. They love their teachers and coaches because these folks are kind and encouraging. As children develop, they learn to give back more and more to the special people they love and who love them. At a certain age they begin to plumb the depths of romantic love. Of course the hormones are raging in those middle school and high school years, but it's not only about sexual desire. Learning how to give and receive love is a huge, huge part of growing up through adolescence. As far as I know the ability to love is innate. We are wired chemically and genetically for affiliation which is one step in the loving process. The modeling of loving parents and extended kin and friendship networks expands that innate ability by teaching the child how to express the many varieties of love that are possible.

Getting back to Jasmine's comment that she's not sure what love is: That is so on-point for a child with Asperger Syndrome. Helen thinks that Jasmine just needs some kind of education to allow the love to flow. However, Jasmine's non-empathetic, black-and-white thinking keeps trying to categorize love as if it were a thing, an object (like a paper weight),

> Jasmine's non-empathetic, black-and-white thinking keeps trying to categorize love as if it were a thing, an object (like a paper weight), something to be acquired. Yet love is a process that changes with each person you love and alters throughout the course of each relationship (like the flow of a mountain stream).

something to be acquired. Yet love is a process that changes with each person you love and alters throughout the course of each relationship (like the flow of a mountain stream). When you compare the two ways of looking at love, it makes sense that concrete-thinking Jasmine is not sure what love is. How could she be when love keeps changing like shifting sand? (Remember we are each a changing individual in a changing world. Our love is a dynamic dialogue with those we love.)

Helen asks a very good question. Can you teach love? I am sure you can, but I doubt that Helen's two children will master the art of love in the same way. While Jason learns from the social milieu, Jasmine has to be instructed step by step. With the rules of engagement we can approximate the skills of loving. Helping Jasmine understand love might be as simple as telling her that there are many different types of love, and then defining each type.

The Greeks define love

Let's try on an example that you might adapt for your own rules of engagement, even though it may sound a might academic. The ancient Greeks define love in four ways, Agápe, Éros, Philia, and Storge. Using these esoteric words with your child may seem a bit "geeky" or contrived. Remember, when a parent is trying to teach his or her Asperger child about the art of love, the more concrete and succinct, the more "geeky" the tools used the better. With these "love" terms in play, the AS child will grow up less confused about love. Add your own new definitions, too. You might even try using the Greek explanations with your AS spouse to help him or her understand that you want to be front and center in the context of their life.

Here are the definitions of love, according to the ancient Greeks. While there are many more nuances in meaning than I have listed, this is enough to get you started guiding your Aspie in the art of love. And yes, you can tell your Aspie that it is possible to have more than one type of love for a person.

Agápe refers to true love. This is the deep and abiding affection one has for one's spouse, partner, or children. It is more than sexual attraction. When we feel Agápe we say, "I love you deeply."

Éros **is passionate and romantic love**. It includes sensuality and longing. Sexual feelings are usually considered a part of Éros. When we feel Éros, we say with much gusto, "I'm crazy about you!"

Philia means friendship. This is the kind of love one has for friends. It is not as passionate as Éros. Philia is displayed with our friends through respect and loyalty and enjoying our time together. Philia is also the type of love we experience when we enjoy an activity. With our friends we might say, "It was great seeing you." Or if we enjoy an activity, we might say, "I just love soccer." We don't love soccer or our friends the way we love our dear ones or our heartthrob.

Storge means affection. It is love, but just of the moment. Within the family where Agápe is strong, a parent will have affection, or Storge, for their child at a moment the child does something adorable. You can have Storge for your pet, but it is probably not on the level of the Agápe you feel for your child.

You don't need a sycophant![36]

Teaching an AS child about the nuances of love may be difficult, but consider the difficulties an NT has co-parenting with his or her Asperger spouse on this topic. The NT thinks of love as the art of loving, or the flow of affection, passion, and a deepening bond in the relationship. The AS co-parent considers love succinct—like a noun, or a thing, incapable of change. While the NT needs verbal and behavioral demonstrations of love to evaluate where the relationship is flowing at the moment, the Aspie is content with knowing in his or her heart that

---

36   A sycophant is a person who uses insincere flattery to win influence from an influential person.

the love is there. No demonstrations needed. Once you got it, you got it. One "I love you" should be enough for a lifetime, according to many Aspies.

As role models for their children, an AS/NT husband and wife will undoubtedly send confusing messages about love and loving. An NT parent might be able to teach the AS child the multiple definitions of love, first promulgated by the ancient Greeks. But how does the NT parent teach the AS child to demonstrate love, to give and receive love—if the AS parent doesn't understand how to reciprocate a loving encounter?

This failure to connect on the part of an AS child or spouse unnerves NT parents and partners, leaving them feeling unloved. This connecting piece is another aspect of empathy. Aspies have a difficult time with empathy, because it requires a different brain organization than they are born with. As we have learned from the theories described in this book, Aspies do not have the brain wiring to create *true* *empathy*, or a true connection. On the other end of the spectrum, NTs are sometimes so connected or "tuned in" to a friend or loved one that they can finish the other person's sentences. Not so with Aspies. You may share with your Aspie many times a certain gesture or word that has deep meaning for you. Still, your Aspie mate may have no comprehension that your intent is a message of love.

Vivian tells this story about her AS husband, Todd. Vivian and Todd are a busy couple with three young children and full time jobs outside the home. Still Vivian is marvelously organized. The house is well kept. She loves to cook, so she prepares nutritious meals for her family each evening. Vivian gardens, too, and scrapbooks with friends. Every Sunday she whisks the children off to church while Todd sleeps in. Vivian loves her life as a mom and wife and community member, because there are many rewards. But she needs Todd, too. When it comes to the messages of love that are so common between partners,

Todd never seems to get the message that Vivian would like some daily demonstration of affection.

One day Vivian is in my office and she says, "Is it really too much to ask of Todd to tell me he loves me?"

I reply, "No, of course it's not too much to ask Vivian. We all need those verbal displays of affection. Obviously you know that Todd loves you, but hearing the words confirms for you that your relationship is still sound. It's like a check-in on the progress of the relationship, because it is bound to change over time. Do you know what I mean?"

"Yes," says Vivian, "I do Dr. Marshack. You've explained Dialectical Psychology and context sensitivity and all that, but Todd is very weird about this stuff. He tells me that he doesn't believe in PDA, public displays of affection. He's okay if we hold hands, but he wouldn't dare give me a kiss in public or, Heaven forbid, say, 'I love you,' in front of others. He rarely says, 'I love you,' at home. And I worry about the children, because Daddy is just not there emotionally. He's kind and a good man and all, but he treats the children like they are adults and should just know that he loves them, too. Todd would never understand that bumper sticker that reads, 'Have you hugged your kid today?'"

Having grown tired of waiting for Todd to tell her he loved her, one day Vivian had prompted him. According to Vivian she hadn't nagged and had used a sweet and gentle tone of voice. "Todd, I love you so much you know."

Todd had said, "Yes, I know."

Vivian had smiled a loving smile at Todd and had tried to get his attention again. "Well I was just wondering if you could tell me you love me, too. You do love me don't you?" Vivian was checking in on their evolving relationship just to be sure they were on track as a romantic couple should be. She couldn't have been more startled by his response.

Todd had turned briefly in Vivian's direction and had asked matter-of-factly, "Why do I need to say that? You don't need a sycophant." Vivian hadn't even known what a "sycophant" was. Todd hadn't been angry, but just before he'd turned to walk away he'd had another thought: "Don't you know you aren't the only woman I could have married?" With that pronouncement, Todd had turned around and walked off to the garage, leaving Vivian bewildered.

"Oh Vivian I am so sorry," I say. "You deserve to be loved and to receive love from your husband. It is so special to have those tender little moments between sweethearts. I hate to be the bearer of bad news, but Todd is not wired for these things. He is wired for the facts. The facts are that he loves you, but he is terrible at demonstrating his love. It's that empathy imbalance hypothesis we talked about. Todd's just stuck in the cognitive side of the equation and *context blind* enough that he is only aware of his own world. Todd thinks because he married you that you should trust his love for you forever—as if love is nothing more than a photo in an album. It is one of the reasons so many NTs complain that, after the wedding, the romance completely disappears from their AS/NT marriage."

"Okay okay. You've told me these things before," Vivian says impatiently. "But tell me this. What on earth is a sycophant? Is that another Aspie totally-made-up word like spousal unit?" Vivian was more curious with than mad at Todd.

I explain, "A sycophant is a 'brown-noser' to use the popular vernacular! They are the kind of people who use compliments or flattery in order to gain advantage with another person."

Vivian cries, "Oh my God! Do you mean to tell me that Todd thinks expressing love for his wife is idle, self-serving flattery? Doesn't he understand even in the remotest part of his Aspie brain that his one-and-only needs a bit of affection once in a while? Please tell me there is a good ending to this story."

"Well of course there's a good ending Vivian," I counter. "It's the same as I've told you before. Both of you need to become experts on Asperger Syndrome. I don't mean the actual diagnosis but how Aspies create Ongoing Traumatic Relationship Syndrome in NTs. They do it unwittingly by saying things like Todd did when he threw out the word, 'sycophant.' When you understand it more, you can apply this knowledge to yourself and your relationship. Knowledge is power. You can create rules of engagement, so that Todd knows better how to tell you he loves you. But you will also need to be satisfied that he does love you— as evidenced by the effort he puts into learning the rules; because he will continue to blunder. I wish I could tell you that Todd will magically develop *true empathy* and intuitively know how to put you in the forefront of his life context, but that won't happen. Instead you must focus on further developing rules of engagement, or behavior guidelines."

Once again an NT is baffled by the pristine logic of an Aspie. If Todd knew about the four types of Greek love, I would anticipate this to be his next response to Vivian's question about whether she is loved: "I thought we went over this already. My feelings are Agápe with a little Éros tossed in." The problem for the Aspie is staying in the flow of the relationship and making "I love yous" a standard part of everyday conversation with their NTs.

Bibliophiles, Lexophiles and Polyamory = Love?

It's interesting that Todd used the word, "sycophant." Number one, he conveyed with one word his belief system about affection. Very efficient and Asperger-like. Number two, he knows this word, and it is a legitimate word. Again very Aspie-like. Todd is well read and absorbs knowledge at a phenomenal rate, because he reads voraciously. Todd, a bibliophile or book lover, taught himself to read when he was in kindergarten and was a fluent reader of chapter books by the time he started first grade. Many with Asperger Syndrome are lexophiles, or lovers of words, and Todd is one of the best. Todd probably has no trouble understanding the concept of Philia as applied to books and words. The question is how to turn that Philial love into Agápe affection for his wife and children.

Another AS/NT couple tells a similar story. Anne Marie was speechless when her AS husband, Tony, asked her to consider a polyamorous lifestyle (more than one sexual partner). It came out of the blue. They got along fine, each managing responsibilities around the house and contributing fairly equally to the household income. A childless couple in their early 40s, they had lots of free time on their hands to do the things they love, such as skiing, traveling, and dining out. Anne Marie enjoyed spending time with her nieces and nephews when she wasn't with Tony. She was a wonderful auntie, who doted on the children, giving them little gifts and taking them on short trips by train to see the local countryside.

Anne Marie was aware that Tony was not the "best" lover. He seemed detached from her when they made love. He couldn't seem to understand that what worked in the bedroom the other day might not work today. There was no variety in his love-making and certainly very little interest in what pleasured Anne Marie. Still she loved him and felt he loved her. Of course she was alarmed when Tony suggested that he needed other intimate relationships.

This crisis brought both of them into therapy. In one session Tony finally reveals the reasoning behind his request for his wife to join him in polyamory. In earnest he explains, "I believe in being open and honest. I love my wife very much, but there is something missing for me. I don't want to break up. Everything works just perfectly for us . . . everything. It's just that I am not head-over-heels in love with Anne Marie. So I thought one way for us to stay together would be to have other sexual friends."

Avoiding the issue of morality and aiming more for the practical side of Tony's suggestion, I say, "That's very logical Tony, but have you considered how these other 'friends' may weaken your ties to Anne Marie?"

Tony says, "Oh I don't think it would hurt. She is free to find other men, too. We just need to be open and honest and have agreements about who we see. And of course the other parties need to have agreements with us, too. I was reading all about it on the Internet. There is a small, but growing 'Poly' community in our area. We could join them and find out the rules." Tony smiles with satisfaction that his plan is so well thought out. Tony was creating his own rules of engagement without consulting Anne Marie—not exactly what is intended by this concept.

Anne Marie comes to Tony's defense before I can respond. By this point Anne Marie has heard all of this many times and isn't as emotionally reactive to Tony. She's even considering trying out the "Lifestyle." She says, "I have known Tony for a long time Dr. Marshack. I believe he does love me, but he doesn't know 'how' to love me. I think he is hoping this will help."

I say, "Thank you Anne Marie. Tony what do you think about what Anne Marie just said? Are you hoping that you will learn more about loving Anne Marie if you investigate polyamory?" I look at Tony and hope we can get past the self-absorption.

"Well it's not exactly like that," says Tony. "I have loved other women, too. But there was only one who I deeply loved. . . and lost. She was my first girlfriend ever. We dated all through high school, but when we went off to college she broke up with me. I never got over that. . . never. And I just don't feel the same about Anne Marie."

Again Anne Marie sits there quietly with a look of compassion on her face. She is well aware that her husband is a lost soul, searching for love and not coming "from" love. She doesn't have the heart to tell

Tony that perhaps he'd lost that girlfriend because he'd been unable to give love back the way NTs need to be loved.

Since Tony is so open and willing I offer this analysis. "Tony, I want you to consider that you have been missing out on love in your marriage and maybe your life because of the way you look at things. Each relationship is so unique that love is never the same between two people. Just as no two people on the planet have the same fingerprints, no two couples love each other the same way. If you expect your love for your wife, Anne Marie, to be exactly like your first love as a teenager, no wonder you don't recognize the deep and abiding love you have for each other. The head-over-heels excitement of young love is not often repeated as we get older. Sure there is excitement in new love relationships, but if that is what you are looking for in a polyamorous life, that is all you will get. As soon as the bloom has faded from the new encounter, you will seek another and another and never really find the deep love you search for."

Tony, like Todd and Jasmine, and many people with Asperger Syndrome, has a difficult time managing the mysteries of a dynamic loving relationship. They can be fascinated by tangible things like their train collection. They can have a love of books and words. They might even be in love with a woman's hair color. But being able to reach out to others with expressions of love that are appropriate for that moment in time—well that is very difficult when empathy is at a minimum.

For Tony, it is very logical to believe that there is only one kind of love between a man and a woman. He believes he is not in love with his wife, because it doesn't feel the same as what he felt for his teenage girlfriend. This black-and-white (and *context blind*) Aspie thinking led Tony to find a solution outside of himself in polyamory. His reasoning is that if he doesn't feel the same about Anne Marie as he felt about his old girlfriend, then the problem is with Anne Marie. Swapping out partners for a new "model" in the hopes that love will be deeper with the next person is a superficial and heartbreaking way to go through life.

No wonder co-parenting within an AS/NT relationship is so difficult. Jasmine, still a teenager, indicated that she isn't sure what love is all about. It appears from Todd and Tony that there are many adults with AS who don't get it either. Whether you and your AS partner have AS or NT children or both, they will be exposed to the most extreme views of love—because of the AS/NT family in which they are reared. Is love a process or an object? Is it what you feel in your heart, or is it how you demonstrate your affection? Is it really love if the other person doesn't acknowledge the emotional gifts you offer or reciprocate them?

Can you teach love? "Maybe," is the best answer I can give you. And it does require the hard work of both partners. Each must be willing to learn and go to therapy in order to develop tools to build an "interface protocol" between the two "operating systems" of neurotypical and Asperger realities.

Lessons learned

1. Love is an innate human experience for Aspies as well as NTs. Don't let yourself believe that Aspies can't love: Because they are *context blind*, their ability to demonstrate love is limited.

2. If you have developed Ongoing Traumatic Relationship Syndrome, it is not too late to reconstruct the love in your AS/NT parenting partnership.

However, you have to get professional help to define the ever-so-important rules of engagement.

3. NT children learn the art of loving from the social milieu by the time they're in preschool, even if they have an Asperger parent. Stop worrying about whether they will adopt your AS partner's style of quantifying love. In order for your NT child to comprehend being loved absent demonstrations of affection, you will have to help him or her adapt to their AS parent.

4. Get your AS spouse on board and go to psychotherapy together. There is no way you can co-parent when your partner has no comprehension about how Asperger's affects the flow of love in the family.

5. Your AS child needs explicit instruction on the art of loving. Love is a mystery for all of us, but for the AS child the mystery is unsolvable without guidance. Use the Greek names for love as a place to start.

6. Know that you are loved, even without verbal and physical demonstrations of affection. When you come from a place of love, you encourage the love to flow.

7. If you come from love—and that means loving yourself, too—then you must make time for yourself. Scrapbook with your friends, sign up for adult league soccer, turn on some music and take a nap—even if it is in the parked car between errands.

CHAPTER ELEVEN

The Power of Intention

In Chapter Six, "The Rules of Engagement," I introduced you to the rules of engagement and explained that their foundation is Dialectical Psychology. In this chapter, I want to help you better understand how to expand those rules. That will enable you to reach more deeply into the mind of your Asperger Syndrome parenting partner and understand his or her intentions. You will learn that "It's not all talk." The rules of engagement are much more than words. They make up a tool that grows with your evolving understanding of and compassion for your Aspie parenting partner.

There is something about these rules that forces us to reframe our perceptions of parenting with an Aspie partner. The rules are a concrete representation of good intentions in the parenting enterprise of your family. Once you "get" that you can't always communicate or relate or parent with Aspies the same way you can with neurotypicals, the whole process becomes easier and less fraught with discord.

I want to draw your attention again to the e-mail from the Aspie husband quoted in the Introduction. He is very aware of the problem of trying to communicate with his spouse when intention—with no verbal or non-verbal outlets for expression—can be so misinterpreted.

> *I've been with my NT partner. . . for 25 years and have inflicted many distressing incidents on her similar to those you describe. But I can honestly say that none of them were ever designed to hurt. This feeling has probably made things much worse for her! I doubt I would have become so angry and defensive if I didn't believe myself to be 'innocent' of the crime of intention. Hopefully I am coming to realise that I need to do more than just not intend to do harm. . . .*

In "Power of Intention," I expand the parenting paradigm by giving examples of specific parenting/partnering techniques compatible with the rules of engagement. I also show you how to express your good intentions in creative and healthy ways. These examples don't form an exhaustive parenting manual; rather they're a representation of the power of intention. You'll see that when you come from a loving heart and an open mind, communicating (and parenting) with your AS spouse (and other family members) can transcend the limits of verbal interaction. That's the place where so many AS/NT couples get locked down.

Doing a 180

One particularly stressful day, my AS daughter, Bianca, went into full meltdown mode. She was 17. Bianca had stood at the top of the stairs by my home office door, screaming that I take care of whatever she was demanding of me. My last clients had been about to leave, so I'd politely excused myself with a comment that even the psychologist has family dilemmas. I'd hoped they would buy this and not hold it against me that my daughter was so out of control.

I'd been exhausted from a long day with my clients, but Bianca had shown me no mercy. She'd raged for a couple of hours. I'd followed her around the house trying to comfort her, trying to understand, but all I'd done was stir it up more. I'd still been a helicopter mother then. Eventually I'd worn out and had just tried to get away from her. I'd gone back to my office and locked the door. But Bianca had begun beating on the door so ferociously that I'd feared she would bruise her hands or break down the door, so I'd opened it. She'd stormed in, continuing to rage. She'd had tears streaming down her face. The snot had been dripping from her nose, and she'd made no attempt to wipe it away even when I'd handed her a tissue. She'd just stood there, making no sense and looking as fierce and frightened as I had ever seen her.

I'd felt my legs weaken underneath me, so I'd reached for my desk chair and sat down. I decided to just sit there and be held hostage for the duration of the siege. I don't really remember what possessed me to take the next action: I noticed my camera sitting next to the computer. I picked it up and began taking pictures of Bianca as she raged at me. I took a couple of pictures of her before she asked me in hostile surprise, "What are you doing?"

At least I had her attention. Stating the obvious I said, "I'm taking your picture." Then Bianca pulled a huge hunk of hair out of her head and screamed louder. I was snapping pictures so fast that I caught this self-abuse in more than one photo.

"Take my picture! I don't care!" she screamed at me, but this time she was at least making sense. So I took more photos.

With each snap of the camera, Bianca came more under control until she finally fell exhausted onto the loveseat. She looked at me very bewildered. Her eyes seemed to be calling out to me for help. Her face was red and swollen. I put the camera down and gingerly handed her a tissue even though I worried this gesture would start her raging again.

Instead she accepted the kindness; then I felt safe to sit next to her on the loveseat and put my arm around her.

I call this intervention, "Doing a 180," because it is an abrupt turnaround that results from doing the opposite of what your Aspie expects. During raging times like this you can try to take a time-out, but I have found that Aspies seldom let you do that. They come after you. You are the object of their distress. You are the source of their distress. You are the solution to their distress. Yet they have no way to express these intentions except to rage at you.

Once you recognize an Aspie's intention, you can relax, detach and take the appropriate 180-degree action. When I picked up the camera, I abruptly changed the course of my daughter's meltdown. I was no longer her object, source or solution. I stepped out of making meaning of her behavior and started the neutral process of recording it with photos. Sensing this change, Bianca calmed down. I think she "got" that I love her and want the best for her even in those moments when she is so out of control. Believe it or not, my 180-degree actions calmed me, too. In my calmer state, I was able to convey another good intention—that I believed Bianca could calm herself down and engage with me in a more appropriate way.

I don't expect you to start taking photos each time you attempt a 180-degree turnaround. Do what makes sense to you. The key is to detach, get to a neutral place, recognize that there is a good intention somewhere underneath all of the confusing communication; then let your intuitive self come up with a strategy. Often what works is the exact opposite of common sense, making it a true 180!

The Universal Translator

I envy those who live on the Federation Starship Enterprise of "Star Trek" fame. They have all of this fascinating space age technology to help them make sense of their environment. One of my most favorite "Star Trek" tools is the Universal Translator. Have you ever wondered why humanoid and not-so-humanoid beings from all parts of the Galaxy (and beyond) are able to talk with each other on the Starship Enterprise? Well, it's because there is a special computer, the Universal Translator, on board the ship. It's this fancy computer's job to translate every language and send the translations directly to the chip implanted in the brain of every officer on the Enterprise. I love it!

Would that we could have had a Universal Translator, so that my AS daughter's wish could have come true: When she was a middle school child, Bianca had wished that people could just read her mind, so that she didn't have to figure out what they wanted.

While a Universal Translator does not exist, we do have another option: Always speak to the good intention, whatever it is, even if you are not sure. When you get a confusing message from your Aspie partner or child, always assume it makes sense somehow, someway. Trust that there is a good intention behind the message even if your partner is speaking Vulcan or Romulan or Ferengi—or Aspie. By maintaining a neutral position, you are better able to answer the question, "Why is he/she telling me this?"

When I get stumped by a confusing message from an Aspie, I use the phrase, "That's right," in order to bring me to neutral. I mentioned this rule in Chapter Six, "The Rules of Engagement." The phrase reminds me that the other person is "right" in that they have a good intention, which has meaning to them. "That's right," also helps me know that I am "right," in that I am capable of good intentions. You may not always be able to get the message translated, but at least being in neutral puts you in a much better frame of mind for the attempt.

Here's a simple example. When Bianca was 8, she wrote me the note you see here. She grew up around my home office, so she observed that my office manager and I often exchanged written notes (even with the advent of e-mail). If I was with a client, Bianca would leave me a note, so that I would be sure to answer her when I had a break from appointments. Notes became Bianca's version of the Universal Translator. The following quote is from the darling little-girl note she wrote me about a problem she was having at school:

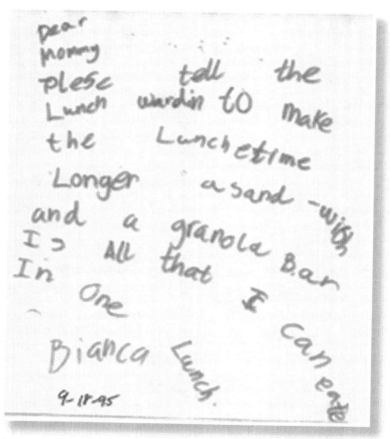

"Dear Mommy Plese tell the Lunch Wardin to make the Lunchtime longer a sand-wich and a granola bar is all that I can eat in one lunch Bianca"

Clearly Bianca was trying to resolve her lunch crisis by asking Mommy to help out. She assumed that I had the super power to expand her lunch time. What mother doesn't love to have this exalted admiration from her child? Furthermore I know that Bianca loves lunch. She loves all meals and snacks. Her goal in the note is to get more time to eat, not eat less.

A couple of days later Bianca used the Universal Translator again. She left me another note about her lunch problem. It read:

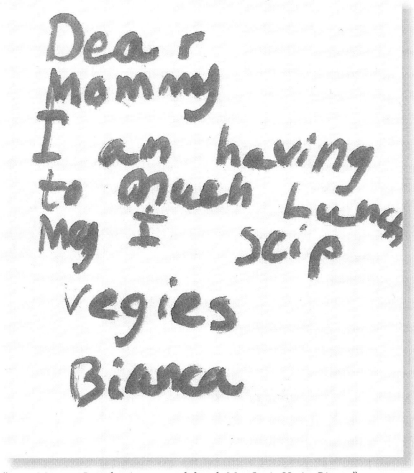

"Dear Mommy I am having to much lunch May I scip Vegies Bianca"

With this second note Bianca had figured out that Mommy does not have the power to lengthen her lunch time. However, she still believes that notes will work. She still believes that Mommy will help.

217

She also believes that she must ask permission to eat less lunch. And it appears she is hoping that she can skip those dreaded "veggies." Bianca's penchant for writing as opposed to talking with me should be noted. It is a typical Aspie trait to find comfort in the written word—because face-to-face communication requires empathy and the interpretation of confusing non-verbal messages.

Bianca's good intentions are obvious, and it is always easier to read between the lines with a young child. The process is no different with an adult. Ask yourself what you know about the person. What is important to him or her? What are their interests, beliefs and opinions? Then do your best to speak to those things, instead of relying only on your interpretation of reality.

Because Aspies have zero degrees of empathy and *context blindness*, their Universal Translator may be writing; because it eliminates the need for them to read nonverbal cues or other aspects of interpersonal context. NTs, on the other hand, have the ability to be more multi-dimensional in their construction of a Universal Translator. I introduced you to Robin (an NT) in Chapter Eight, "Bullied or Bully?" Robin discovered that using her Universal Translator made it much easier to understand and eventually let go of her former husband, Aldo, an Aspie. At least the understanding the Universal Translator provided made it easier for Robin to resolve the divorce crisis—the painful puzzle of her husband's abusive behavior. The following is a short dialogue I had with Robin one day.

"Dr. Marshack I have been so hurt for years by something that Aldo wrote to me in an email when we were divorcing." Robin's expression seems to indicate that she has an idea she wants to run by me.

"Go ahead Robin. What are you thinking?" I prompt.

Robin continues, "Well in one of our first divorce court hearings I was deeply troubled that Aldo was fighting me over temporary child support. Previously he told me that he wanted to help with everything for the children so that they wouldn't suffer because of our divorce, especially the tutors for our two ASD [Autism Spectrum Disorder] kids. But at the hearing, his attorney told the judge that I was lying about the children's financial needs and convinced the Judge to cut in half what I asked for. I was stunned because I knew Aldo could afford more, even with a separation. I sat in the courtroom and cried."

I nodded my support for how painful this experience had to be for Robin. My hint of a smile encourages Robin to continue her train of thought. "When I got home I wrote Aldo an e-mail about my disappointment. I explained that I was deeply hurt that he would pull such a trick and leave his family in the lurch. I couldn't fathom his callousness, especially since I believe that he really loves his children. But Dr. Marshack, his response to this e-mail has kept me stuck and miserable for years. Do you know what he said?"

Robin looks at me for more approval that it's okay to finally resolve this problem. I give it, "No Robin, I can't imagine what he said, but I bet it makes sense to you now, doesn't it?"

Robin is encouraged. "Yes it does Dr. Marshack, but it felt so awful at the time. Aldo had written back and said, 'You're just mad because I won.' Until I started using the Universal Translator, I was left feeling anguish over this response. I felt like I had been horribly betrayed. I mean, how could Aldo possibly think our children were to be used like that in a zero-sum game of win-lose? But recently I have been rethinking that e-mail. I've realized that Aldo was just so emotionally overwhelmed that he couldn't say what was really in his heart."

I think Robin is asking for some feedback from me, so I start to opine about Aldo's intention behind his remark. But before I can say anything, Robin stops me. She looks at me as if to read my mind and says, "Yes I know what you are thinking. I figured it out myself. The reason I felt so betrayed by Aldo's comment is that he was feeling betrayed by me. I was the one who filed for divorce. I am sure he never thought in a million years that I would leave him. So he felt betrayed and confused by my actions and decided he couldn't trust me about anything, even how much money I needed to care for our children. Instead of really analyzing the numbers, he'd just assumed that I was lying and that he had to fight me. It is very sad isn't it? But now I feel free of the pain of thinking Aldo is a monster who'd wanted to win more than do the right thing for his children. He'd just felt betrayed, and I wish he would accept my apology."

I look at Robin with a bit of doubt in my expression, and she picks up on it right away.

"Oh Dr. Marshack! I am not blaming myself, not at all!" she exclaims adamantly. "I still think what Aldo did was immature and unconscionable. To try to strangle me financially just to get even, well that was just wrong, especially when we still had kids to raise. But I do understand better why he did it. It's a relief to realize that it was just an Aspie thing."

While Robin's analysis may seem complex or even irrationally skewed to some of you, it is not a bad interpretation of Aldo's actions. After all she'd lived with him for many years, and he'd never demonstrated a serious lack of conscience until he wrote that e-mail. Because of Aldo's empathy disorder, he didn't understand that his wife could still love him and leave him—and that in the process of a divorce she could still be trusted. What Robin figured out, finally after many years, is that Aldo's feelings of betrayal got translated into behavior designed to betray Robin. Her "stuckness," or unresolved feeling of betrayal, was telling her to look at the feeling as a reflection of what Aldo was feeling but could never speak.

It is ironic that Aldo's empathy disorder handicapped Robin, too. Because Aldo could not properly connect words with his feelings of betrayal, he stumped Robin in her process of recovering from the divorce. While Robin may never get a chance to clear up the mystery with Aldo, her new understanding of the "Aspie thing," will enable her to feel free to move on with her life.

The Universal Translator can be used for something as simple as recognizing your child's need for help with a school lunch problem or something as intense and complex as a divorce betrayal. It is a matter of recognizing that the other person's behavior makes sense to them— even if they are using a language you may not understand. Once you accept this, you are in a better position to connect with your Aspie's good intention, even if the behavior is confusing or abusive.

Don't fix it

One powerful type of intervention is to stop trying to fix him/her or you or it. It may seem like codependency to accept that your Aspie partner needs you to handle lots of the organizational things that elude them. Hannah found that things went much better with Raphael when she wrote down everything— and I do mean everything. She wrote her thoughts in e-mails and texts. She wrote paper letters and slipped them into his briefcase to read later. She made lists of items for Raphael to buy at the grocery store, replete with the brand name and price. This method gave Raphael time to consider what his wife was telling him and to sort for her good intentions. The fact that Raphael wanted to read her notes was evidence to Hannah that he loved her and was responding to her good intentions, too.

In spite of her patience with her husband's need for notes, Hannah got unnerved when Raphael insisted on Post-it notes as yet another method for writing it down. She didn't mind if he wrote the notes to himself. What bothered her was that he wanted her to write him notes on Post-its, so that he could stick them places as reminders. Raphael placed pads of Post-it notes in his pockets and in his car; then deposited them in convenient locations throughout the house, even the bathroom. Hannah got used to finding Raphael's Post-it notes attached to mirrors, closet doors, books, tools, the car visor, inside his coat, even stuck to his cell phone. But she resisted writing the notes for him. Each time he asked her to do so, she complained that he could do it himself.

One day I confront Hannah. "Hannah it's true that you don't have to write the Post-it notes for Raphael, but have you thought about why he asks? I mean, there may be a kind of logic to it. What do you think?"

Hannah looks at me with wide-eyed amazement. She says, "Nope I won't do it. I do everything for him already. He would forget to get gas or brush his hair or get milk at the store or take our children to the wrong park for soccer practice. . . if it weren't for me. He wouldn't even show up to work on time if I didn't remind him that it was time to get out the door. Nope I help him stay on task for all kinds of things, and I write him emails and texts already, so why do I have to do one more inane thing like write Post-it notes for him?"

I say, "Well, it might just be that Raphael is more motivated to re-member if you write the Post-it note."

Hannah stops shaking her head and looks at me with interest. "Okay" she says, "What do you mean?"

"It's like this," I continue. "Remember when we discussed that Aspies have zero degrees of empathy and also have *context blindness*?" Hannah nods in the affirmative. "So what this means is that they have to use other devices for remembering things. They don't have those subtle internal signals that warn them they are about to fall asleep, or how much time it will take to finish their shower and get off to work, or how to remember those little things that the rest of us can organize in our minds. Remember they are *context blind*. So instead of intuition to guide them through the maze of multiple competing priorities, they of-ten rely on external structure—rigid structure—to keep them on target.

One of Raphael's systems, or structures, is to use Post-it notes to jog his memory about everything."

Hannah says sarcastically, "Yeah, I get it. But why do I have to write the note for him. . .when he has a pen in his hand and a pad of Post-its in his pocket?" Hannah is exasperated with me but she still trusts that I might have an idea she has yet to think of.

I continue, "Here's my supposition about his good intentions. First, Raphael wants you to write the Post-it notes, because it is confirmation that you approve of his system and don't see it as foolish. Besides you write all of the other notes. . . e-mails, texts and letters. In other words, it is a system you reinforce every time you write a note for your husband. Second, he may worry that he won't word it correctly and will make some silly mistake like come home with canned tuna when you requested canned salmon. Remember, he is *context blind*, so he doesn't read non-verbal cues very well at all. Third, I wonder if a note in your handwriting helps him associate the task with you, someone he loves and wants to help. I don't know, I could be wrong, and we would have to ask him, but what do you think?"

Hannah is amused. "What on earth? This makes sense. Poor guy. He doesn't know how to explain why he keeps handing me the Post-its even though I tell him all the time that I don't want to write them for him. It makes me feel like I'm his mother. But now that you explain it this way it makes so much sense. What a terrible burden he must carry that he can't remember anything without all kinds of prompts. Then he finally finds a nutty little system that seems to work for him, like the Post-its, and I come along and trash it. I guess I just wanted to fix him again!"

I look Hannah squarely in the eye and ask her, "What about my notion that your handwriting triggers his love for you and his desire to please you? Have you ever considered that he loves you even with all of the organizing and reminding you have to do for him? It just might be that you forgot the love that brought you two together in the first place—because, well you are filled with resentment about the extra work he requires."

Hannah tears up a bit and nods her head. "Yes you are so right Dr. Marshack. I let my distress and fatigue get the best of me. If I can just remember that Raffi is a devoted, loving, hard-working husband and father. . . and if I can see the things I do for him as stuff that he needs to manage the limitations imposed by his AS. . . well then it's not about fixing him, or being irritated. . . it's about just loving him. I like that. Thank you for hanging in there with me."

I confirm Hannah's realization. "And Hannah. It's not about fixing you either. You are good at reading people and the environment. You are good at organizing a busy household and juggling all of the responsibilities smoothly. Be who you are and give that gift to Raphael. In turn he can gift you with the many talents he has."

Disney magic

Animated Disney movies appeal to young and old, because of the imaginative way the story is portrayed on the screen. The music and lyrics are especially memorable, because they are designed to elicit emotions. The characters are not necessarily fully developed, but they are still designed to capture our hearts. The animal characters are especially endearing, because of their innocence about the world. So what is the appeal? What draws us in? Childhood desires and beliefs. Somehow we want to believe that we can go back and capture the innocent spirit of youth, where everything always has a happy ending—or should have.

We grow up and become more sophisticated about the realities of life on Planet Earth. However, there might be value in capturing a bit of the Disney magic to sprinkle on your AS/NT family. I have met many Aspies who are great artists, poets, storytellers and musicians. While Aspies have zero degrees of empathy, mind blindness, and *context blindness*—and while they struggle with creating organization or tracking time—they seem to have an uncanny ability to synthesize an awareness of the world through the arts. I suggest relying on this tool even more with your AS parenting partner.

Caitlynn and her Aspie partner, Sean, were remodeling their home one summer. The tile guys were coming the next day to tile the shower and tub area. Caitlynn knew exactly what she wanted. Sean didn't care what she chose in the way of color schemes or materials as long as she stayed in the budget. But tomorrow was important, because Caitlynn could not stay home to supervise the workers. She was driving one child to day camp at the local park and recreation center. Then she had to swing by band camp with the other child. Before she went to work, she had to pick up a birthday cake for a coworker. It was supposed to be a surprise, so she had to slip it into the lunch room early before her friend could see it. Whew! It was going to be a busy morning.

Sean had offered to help with the juggling act by staying home from work and meeting the tile guys. It was clear to Caitlynn that she couldn't rely on Sean to handle the kids that day and make it back home in time to meet the tile people. And it wasn't practical for him to pick up the cake and deliver it to her workplace. Besides he would probably blow the surprise. So when she analyzed the multiple competing demands, she decided to take a chance that Sean could handle the responsibility of supervising the tiling—but not without some Disney magic.

That evening, as the kids were in the family room playing games, she'd started a discussion with Sean to be sure he understood what she wanted in the bathroom.

"Of course I know what you want honey!" Sean had smiled at her.

"Well Sean it's just that I want to make sure they don't tile over the little spaces in the sheetrock that are for the shampoo and other shower stuff. You know, where I drew the lines on the sheetrock for the shelves?" Caitlynn had done her best to explain what she wanted.

"Oh sure. I know what you mean." Sean had looked confident, but he'd been distracted by the baseball game he was watching.

Caitlynn determined that a little Disney magic would help. She chose a visualization exercise to help Sean better comprehend the situation. "Sean Honey. I know we talked about this, but would you mind playing along with me? You know me, I just get so worried over little things. I want to make sure that everything goes well tomorrow, so that we don't have to tear it out if they goof. I know you can handle it, but would you mind doing a little mind exercise with me?" Caitlynn didn't want to offend Sean, but she was not certain that he had the visual concept of what she wanted.

Sean agreed to turn off the game for a few minutes while Caitlynn walked him through the "mind exercise." She started by asking Sean to close his eyes and imagine the bathroom as it currently was. "Do you see the green waterproof sheetrock on the walls in the tub enclosure?" she asked.

"Yes," said Sean.

"Okay then, and do you see the lines on the sheetrock for the shampoo and toiletries shelves?" she asked.

"Sure," said Sean, and he started to open his eyes.

"No we're not done yet Honey. Please close your eyes again," Caitlynn said gently.

Sean obliged.

Caitlynn continued. "Now I want you to start the process of tiling the bathtub. Imagine that you are picking up one of those new pink tiles we picked out for the bathroom. Can you see them?"

Sean nodded his head.

"Okay Sweetie. Pretend you put glue on the back of the tile and that you place it in the far left corner of the bathtub wall, right next to the tub. Make sure it's in the bottom corner. Have you got it?" Caitlynn was patiently guiding Sean through the process of tiling.

Sean nodded again. "Okay, I put it there. Now what?"

"Okay, so now take another pink tile and place it next to the first one to start a row across the bottom of the wall next to the tub. Is that working for you Sean?"

"Sure I have a whole row of them now," said Sean.

"Great," exclaimed Caitlynn. She was very pleased that Sean was willing to humor her with this little exercise. "Now imagine that you are starting a second row, just above the first one. . . ."

Before Caitlynn could finish describing the process, Sean interrupted her. "No problem Hon. I just tiled up the whole bathtub enclosure! Ha! Oooops! I tiled over the shampoo shelves!" Sean's eyes had popped open and with a laugh he'd said to Caitlynn, "Gotta make sure those tile guys don't make the same mistake."

Granted, this bit of Disney magic is not very sophisticated or entertaining, but the basic principles can be applied to any situation. Engage the mind in a fantasy (using one or several senses) in order to create meaning. It works for all types of creative expression whether in the arts or a conversation between life/parenting partners, who are remodeling their home. This technique seems to break through the barriers imposed by lack of empathy or context sensitivity.

Many Aspies have figured out that the arts open up a type of creative communication they otherwise would not experience. It can be art as light as a sprinkling of Disney magic or as rich and complex as a symphony performance. Terry, a devout Catholic and an Aspie, lamented that he was not sure he really had a relationship with God. He worried that others talked about this very personal experience with a kind of intensity that escaped him. He wanted what they described, but for some reason his theological education was no help in creating the heart connection he longed for. Until the day when I asked Terry about his experience singing in the church choir. As he'd described the experience, I'd noticed his body shift and his facial expression soften. He'd said, "There's something about singing with the choir that makes me feel inspired."

"Terry, is it possible that this feeling of inspiration is what others describe as a relationship with God?" I ask, looking hopefully at him.

"Maybe." Terry is cautious, because this problem is so sad for him. He wants to really know God, to be one with God, but none of the words in the Bible have led him to this experience. "I do feel the vibrations in my body when I sing. And when I sing with others, I feel their vibrations, too. Sometimes I am even brought to tears by the beauty and majesty of it all. But is that what everyone else is talking about?"

Terry looks at me for the answers to his questions— an enormous task for me. I didn't want to let him down. I didn't want to give him a trite answer—not about God. Terry would know if I was just being philosophical as opposed to really sympathizing with his problem. "Terry I can't speak with certainty that I know what others feel when they describe their relationship with God. I know that people for thousands of years have talked, written, sung, and danced about this special connection, so it must be possible to experience it one way or another. But do you want to know what I think and feel about this God connection you are after?"

Terry seems to appreciate that I am trying, so he nods approval for me to continue.

"Well I believe that we are all connected to each other through God. That means that if you feel joyful and inspired when you are singing, that is a relationship with God or a God moment. Even more phenomenal is that you recognize your connection to others in the choir through the physical vibrations of their singing bodies. Enjoy the moment. But like all such moments our God "realization" doesn't last. It comes and goes as we navigate the roller coaster ride here on Planet Earth."

I am not sure that Terry fully accepts my explanation, but he has helped me better comprehend the power of intention. Whatever the language, God speaks to us and through us. We are all connected and need to be respectful of this connection regardless of our differences—or we may miss God's message.

Ping

Computer metaphors are a marvelous way to help Aspies understand how to empathically communicate with their parenting partner and children. No one has yet built a computer that can compete with the human brain's ability to integrate multiple dimensions of consciousness; however the step-by-step algorithm logic that drives computers has a strong appeal to Aspies. The kind of "computer logic" preferred by Aspies won't necessarily resolve *context blindness* or zero degrees of empathy. It can create opportunities to see that an Aspie has good intention.

In my previous book I told the story of one of my Aspie clients who came to understand that he and his wife think differently and process information differently, much like computers with different operating systems. I'd been delighted by this awareness and had asked my client if there was a solution to create communication between their two operating systems. He'd happily offered that he and his wife needed to build an "interface protocol."

Another of my Aspie clients (a software engineer) used the computer metaphor, pinging, to enhance his understanding of empathic connecting. Alec had perked up when I'd suggested he seek a computer metaphor to better understand his wife. "So Dr. Marshack, are you suggesting that when Hildy interrupts me with a silly question like 'Watcha up to?' that she is just getting my attention. I mean, she isn't really asking what I am doing since she can clearly see I'm at the computer?"

I answer, "Yes Alec. That is exactly what I am saying. Hildy is trying to connect with you. She's just checking in. For NTs, this is a way to say, 'I love you.' And when she says, 'Watcha up to?' she really just wants you to stop what you are doing and acknowledge that she is there. She wants to know that she is more important to you than your computer game. But it doesn't mean she is really asking you what you are doing. She just wants you to stop for a moment, smile at her and say, 'Hello,' or 'Hi Honey.' Does this make sense Alec?"

"Well," Alec offers, "it sounds like pinging to me." Noting the confused look on my face, Alec offers to show me on my laptop. "Let me show you on your computer." He says, "Go to 'Programs' and click 'Accessories.' " I fumble a bit since I am a digital dinosaur.

> Computer metaphors are a marvelous way to help Aspies understand how to empathically communicate with their parenting partner and children. . . .
> "Hildy must feel frustrated when she pings me, and I send her the response 'timed out' or 'host not found'. I think I can do better. . . ." adds Alec

"Alec would you like to show me? I get a bit confused about all of the computer commands." I push the laptop in his direction and Alec takes over.

"Well you click here on 'Accessories,' and then you click on 'Command Prompt.' Then you type the word 'ping.' After that you enter the target website you want to check in with or ping." I still look confused, but Alec is patient. He offers, "Well let's try CNN." As Alec sends the ping, we get an immediate response,

"Request timed out." Alec says, "Oh yeah, we took too long. Let's try again."

"Can we try [pinging] Dr. Carol Markovics? She's a friend of mine."[37] I prompt Alec, and he obliges. We get a response right back, "Ping request could not find host Carol Markovics. Please check the name and try again."

Alec says, "Let me try CNN again, and this time I'll just send the ping instead of talking." Alec enters the command, and immediately we get a response from CNN as the server starts to download code— none of which I can read.

"Well, Alec I think you are on to something," I say. "It appears that pinging is a message that one computer sends to another just to check in. It's a hello message, but there is no attempt to talk about anything in particular. One computer is checking to see if the other computer is awake and responding. After that you have to send other messages if you really want to communicate. Do I have that right Alec?"

He answers, "That's about right Dr. Marshack. So when Hildy drops by my office and says 'Watcha doing?' she's pinging. I can handle that." Alec smiles at his wife.

Hildy is chuckling about the whole thing. She enjoys her husband's sense of humor and is very pleased that he is coming to recognize the good intention behind her "pings."

I continue the metaphor. "So Alec I also want you to notice that sometimes when you ping you get a message that the other computer is not available, such as the message 'timed out' or 'ping request could not find host.' How did you feel when you got those messages? Were you a little frustrated?"

"Oh yea," answers Alec, "I got you Dr. Marshack. Hildy must feel frustrated when she pings me but I send her the response 'timed out' or

---

37 Dr. Carol Markovics is a psychologist specializing in Autism Spectrum Disorders in Portland, Oregon.

'host not found.' I think I can do better. Even when I don't really under-stand why she is asking me stuff, I can assume it is a ping," adds Alec.

I smile at both Hildy and Alec. "Yes I think you've got it Alec. Hildy loves you and sends you pings to find out if you love her, too. Responding to her ping will be easier than you thought won't it?"

Even if your Aspie is a digital dinosaur like me, he or she might ap-preciate this metaphor. It is a simple way to describe one subtlety of NT communication. NTs are always sending and receiving pings. It's a non-verbal method of connecting to their friends and family mem-bers and even strangers at the grocery store. Each ping (or connection) confirms that we are all in this life together. I have found it a powerful metaphor in therapy. You might try it.

It's not all talk

Often those faced with the greatest challenges make discoveries that others miss. Parenting with a partner with Asperger Syndrome is one of those challenges. It provides a great opportunity to expand our consciousness and our creativity. I have offered you lots of information about theories and techniques, but what seems the most important to understand is the power of intention. AS/NT parents are navigating territory that appears at times to be a wild frontier. They have to make it up as they go. The theories presented in this book will help you. The rules of engagement can be a guide. Remember, so many of the parent-ing techniques that work in other families don't work when parenting with an Aspie. What does work: When you believe that we are all con-nected, no matter our differences, and when you seek the good inten-tions. With this approach, you will find more peace in your unusual parenting journey.

Lessons learned

1. The power of intention means that there is strength in "meaning well" when you communicate with your partner.

2. The rules of engagement are a guide and are much more than words. Don't just create and enforce the rules. Think about how to use them to identify the intentions of your AS or NT partner. This helps foster effective parenting.

3. "Doing a 180" is a technique to help you detach from a communication that is emotionally out of control. While keeping good intention in mind, turn to a behavior that is the total opposite of what is expected by the raging Aspie. This has a way of surprising and immediately shutting down the emotionally dysregulated person.

4. The "Universal Translator" is a tool that helps you recognize the intention of the other person. The purpose of the Translator is to help you speak to your partner's good intentions instead of to their confusing behavior. Since this technique requires the ability to put feelings into words in a way that is empathic, it is probably better suited to the NT parent.

5. Use the phrase, "That's right," as a reminder to break out of your "stuck place." Then use any of the other tools that seem appropriate at the moment. This phrase implies—hence generates the feeling—that

you are "right" and the other person is "right," too. It's a means of bringing your good intentions together.

6. "Don't fix it" infers that it is best for parenting partners to work with each other just as they are. If your AS partner likes to use Post-it notes as an external tool to jog his memory and keep him on task, just accept it. This doesn't mean we can't change; but trying to change your partner to be more like yourself seldom works. Instead search for the good intention behind problematic AS behaviors.

7. "Disney magic" is a fanciful term for recognizing that we are all connected in ways beyond intellectual/rational communication. Use movies, music, art, visualization exercises or any other creative means to convey your message. Don't be stuck because your words aren't enough.

8. "Ping" is a computer term that describes the method that NTs use to connect—for no other reason than to connect. Those with Asperger Syndrome often understand this metaphor, so I suggest you use it. Even if your Aspie struggles with empathy, he or she does want to connect and feel the love. Computer metaphors give them a framework and logic to comprehend the subtle meaning of NT communication. Responding to the NT's pings is yet another way an Aspie can demonstrate good intention.

CHAPTER TWELVE

Conclusion: A New Agenda

When my NT daughter, Phoebe, turned 22 and celebrated the 22nd anniversary of her adoption day a month later, she posted on Facebook her feelings about the day. She wrote:

22 years ago today I was adopted into a family that has now fallen apart. The only person left is my mother, my hero & I couldn't be more grateful to have her as my mom.

Sadly Phoebe's sentiments are the inspiration for this book. Too many AS/NT couples and families struggle to the point of the family falling apart—because they have no help to unravel the strange dialectic of Asperger/neurotypical relationships.

I hope that your ride on the roller coaster of *Out of Mind - Out of Sight* has stirred up more than grief over lost years with your loved ones. I hope that the book has inspired you to create a new agenda for parenting with your AS spouse/partner. I hope this new agenda includes: being true to yourself; speaking out about what you believe in; and protecting yourself and your children from abuse. Most of all, I hope it helps you find creative ways to express and recognize the loving intentions deep within all of us—even *context blind* AS family members.

To connect or be destroyed

In the "Introduction," I shared an e-mail I'd received from a man with Asperger's who expressed hope for his marriage after reading my book *Going Over the Edge?* In a few paragraphs he summed up the two major Aspie issues exemplified in this second book, intention and *context blindness*. Please read a portion of his e-mail again below. Imagine the angst this man was feeling, because his good intentions were concealed by his *context blindness* (i.e. "I would be destroyed"). And yet there is hope in his statement, because he believes there is something even greater than his or his wife's good intentions.

> . . . *Reading your [first] book I think I see parallels here between my fear of being overwhelmed in social or conflict situations. But I also see similarities to those feelings when my partner expresses her frustrations and needs—to admit to her point of view seems sometimes like I would be 'destroyed'. I mention this because I get the strong feeling that you equate spirituality and loving relationships. I feel that between myself and. . . there is something very important to us both, beyond companionship. For me there seems to have been a chance given that I would never [have] believed I would have had. . . .*

The dilemma for Aspies is their fear of being destroyed if they connect. To an NT this seems preposterous: Connection is so elementary to us. It is how we come to know ourselves, through our connections with others. We lose nothing of ourselves by connecting and understanding and supporting each other. Just as Klaus Riegel suggests in

Dialectical Psychology, we are comfortable with being "changing individuals in a changing world." We give ourselves over to others every day from the moment we are born to our last breath. But for the Aspie, this reciprocal identification with others is like death, and they fight mightily against it.

Two examples may help you to better comprehend why Aspies choose this defense mechanism. Fifteen-year-old Ramon expresses it well when he says, "I have to have all of the answers, and I have to have the last word, or if I don't, I will be ashamed of myself." Ramon, like most Aspies, is not a team player. He does not learn from others. He does not problem solve with others either. In his arrogant, controlling, obsessive way, Ramon believes he must figure everything out on his own or die trying. Because of his lack of empathy and his *context blindness*, Ramon is not wired to process the cues that others give him. He literally believes he has no choice but to do it all himself: In other words, "Out of Mind - Out of Sight."

Eight-year-old Sasha describes it in yet another way. He calls it lack of flexibility. Sasha is delightful and very bright. He loves drawing maps of the world with all of the climate zones properly color coded. One day in my office he decides to play with the alphabet blocks to create a word search puzzle. Within 10 minutes, he literally uses every letter, except for Q, to create words forwards, backwards, vertically and diagonally—even backwards and diagonally!

Sasha is overly dependent on this and other exceptional Aspie traits, because of his inability to respond appropriately to non-verbal cues—even when the cue is something as loud as the sound of a chain saw. For example, one day loggers were sawing down trees next to my office. Sasha and I looked out the window and watched the loggers for a few minutes. Since Sasha seemed thrilled by the event, I asked if he wanted to go outside on my deck and watch for awhile. He eagerly agreed since he also loves John Deere equipment like the loggers were using. However, when we stepped outside, Sasha looked straight ahead instead of in the direction of the chain saws. The sound was deafening, but he could not determine that the sound was coming from the west until I nudged him to turn in that direction. Remember, Sasha had already looked out my window at the loggers, but now he couldn't orient his body to the sound or sight of the loggers. Nor could he remember having seen their location through the window.

Not only does Sasha lack flexibility when it comes to sensory awareness, but he identified that he and his NT father struggle in this regard. Similar to Ramon, Sasha lacks the flexibility to let go of a subject. Sasha and his father argue and grow frustrated because of this.

It is so very important for us to understand this inflexibility and the shame and fear of being destroyed that fuel Aspies to get through life. Without understanding on both the AS and NT sides, the entire family can fail. I recall reading a couple of newspaper stories that are shocking. In one case a 28-year-old Aspie man was lost for over a month in the Utah desert when he attempted to hike alone for 30 miles. Although he was near well-travelled trails and could have asked people for help, he wandered around lost. It is a miracle that he was found alive.[38] In another, even more tragic, story a 28–year-old Aspie was murdered by his mother, who then turned the gun on herself. The mother left a note at the scene taking responsibility for the murder/suicide. She had previously confided in friends that life with her son was exceedingly hard.[39] What both of these stories show is how out of control and dangerous *context blindness* can be. They illustrate how imperative it is to understand the AS/NT dialectic. *Context blindness* can put someone in physical danger. It can cause the death of relationships, too. We owe it to our Aspie loved ones to help them with this huge limitation—if they will let us.

---

[38] "Utah rescuers find emaciated hiker after month-long ordeal." July 14, 2012. www.cnn.com/2012/07/13/us/utah-desert-rescue/index.html?hpt=us_c1

[39] "Donations sought for Kennewick murder victim." Sept. 30, 2011. www.tri-cityherald.com/2011/09/30/1661904/donations-sought-for-kennewick.html.

Awe-inspiring Aspies

The upside of *context blindness* is the sweet, naïve, sensitivity that we often see in our Aspie loved ones. How is it possible that they can be so tuned in emotionally one minute and so out of touch the next? My daughter Bianca demonstrated this sensitivity so often. On one occasion the family had made a visit to a dying elderly relative, Bianca's great grandmother, "Tutu," a Hawaiian name for grandmother. Bianca had been about 5, and her younger sister, Phoebe, had been about 2. When we'd walked into the nursing home, Phoebe had begun hanging on me as she'd nervously absorbed the sights and sounds of this strange place. Bianca had marched confidently ahead even though she hadn't known where she was going. When we'd gotten to Tutu's room, Bianca had seen the old woman slumped in a wheelchair. She'd boldly walked over to Tutu and had taken her hand. Then Bianca had looked back at Phoebe, who'd been stubbornly refusing to walk past the open door. With Tutu's hand in hers, Bianca had waved her other hand in Phoebe's direction, beckoning her to come in. Bianca had said these reassuring words, "It's okay Phoebe. She's just an 'old one.' "

This sensitivity seemed so amazing to me, but was it really so sensitive? True, Bianca had had no fear of an "old one." In truth, I doubt she'd even known who Tutu was. She had seen her no more than a couple of times since Tutu lived out of state.

Bianca had missed a lot of the contextual clues during that visit. She'd walked into a building she had never been in before and had just marched ahead of her parents without any clear idea of where she was going. Her sensory system had not picked up the sights and smells and sounds that are so characteristic of a nursing home where people are very ill or dying. She hadn't noticed my hesitation at Tutu's door either. When I'd seen Tutu slumped over in the wheelchair, I'd moved slowly so as not to awaken her: I'd also wondered if she was dead. But Bianca had abruptly walked up to Tutu and taken her hand. Had she been aware that Tutu was her great grandmother? Had she truly been supportive of Phoebe's feelings? Or was she simply curious about an "old one?"

Within a year or so of Tutu's death, my own father passed away from a lingering illness. At the funeral I'd asked a friend to give each guest a white carnation as they arrived. I'd expected people to take the carnations home since there was not to be a burial. My father's body lay in a room next door to the chapel. Cremation would follow the funeral, so there was no intention of having a formal casket viewing at the memorial service. We only decided at the last minute to allow people to follow the tradition of paying their last respects by viewing the body. After the funeral, I'd stayed to say goodbye to all of the guests. When the last person was out the door I'd decided to visit my father one last time. I was shocked to enter the room and see his body covered with white carnations. A friend of mine, who had known my father for many years, was still in the room, too. She saw the look of surprise on my face and explained that after the funeral, little 6-year-old Bianca had walked quietly out of the chapel to the viewing room. She'd reverently placed her carnation on my father's body. The other guests had followed Bianca to the room and, one by one, they'd followed her example until the body was covered with white carnations.

I can't explain this away as simply as I can the experience with Tutu. Bianca did know her grandfather very well since we lived close to each other. We celebrated birthdays and holidays together and had regular visits. There was something wiser, and deeper, than curiosity, in Bianca's actions at my father's funeral.

How is it possible that those with *context blindness* and zero degrees of empathy can be so aware of the spiritual nature? Below is a drawing Bianca made when my father was dying in the hospital. She knew something that she could only express through her art. The childish drawing has an unimaginable wisdom. Bianca drew my father in bed with his head lower than his feet. She colored his body black and drew a black smile on his face. All of this is classic symbolism for death. The bed is floating in a sea of radiant sun-washed color. Over

> But what do you do when you have a strong need to express the depth of your emotions but are not sure of the context to do so?

the bed is a cloud with a touch of blue. Above the cloud is a golden heavenly figure looking down over my father. We are not a deeply religious family. We rarely go to church or synagogue even for a holiday, so Bianca did not have much in the way of religious education. Yet at the age of 5, going on 6, Bianca connected with the spirit that guides and connects all of us. On the back of her drawing she wrote a loving message to her grandfather in orange and gold crayon, "Bianca . . . I luv u." Bianca asked me to give the drawing to her grandfather, and it hung in his room until his death.

Many NTs tell me similar stories of the awe-inspiring wisdom of their Aspies. These NT parents/partners are bewildered when they read that Aspies lack empathy or have *context blindness*. But it makes sense just the same. We are all human beings and we all feel connected, but we don't all have the same ability to share that connection with others. If you're an NT and have context sensitivity and strong empathy skills you can verbalize with others and you can sense just what needs to be verbalized. But what do you do when you have a strong need to express the depth of your emotions but are not sure of the context to do so? Well, if you are a 5-year-old AS child, who loves her grandfather very much, and who has tremendous creative ability, you might just draw a picture of what is in your heart.

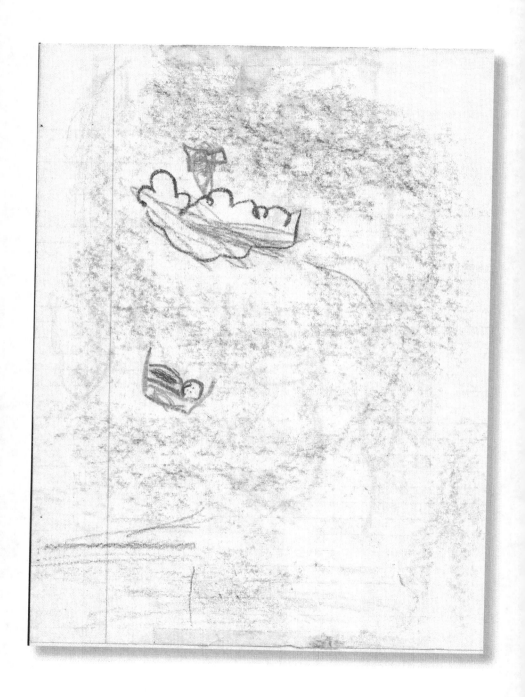

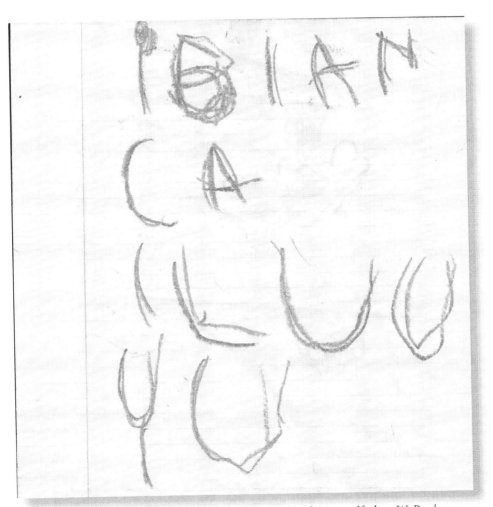

Bianca drew the picture at left in the fall of 1992 when her grandfather, W. Paul Johnson, was near death at Providence Hospital in Portland, Oregon. She was almost 6 years old. Grandpa lived until January 13, 1993. Bianca knew at an intuitive level that her grandfather did not have much time to live-but that he was in good hands. The above words were written on the back of the drawing.

The "Aspie Class" and the "NT Class"

One of my Aspie clients with a great sense of humor has invented a scientific nomenclature to categorize types of human beings. He says he belongs to the "Aspie Class" of human being and that his wife belongs to the "NT Class." Because of his Aspie penchant for coining terms and phrases, we frequently joke about developing a book on the subject. But I have to say there is more than humor in these designations. If you think about it, the terms, "Aspie Class" and "NT Class" are a terrific simple and neutral way to point out the differences between AS and NT loved ones. No judgment; just fact. It is with greater understanding of each class that NTs and Aspies can find common ground in "mixed-class" parenting.

Throughout this book I have attempted to educate parents who have AS partners about the minefields of this mixed-class family life. I hope you come away with some recognition of opportunities to be more successful parents. Still, it is clear that this life is not easy. Many marriages fail under the pressures of mixed-class family life. My own life is no exception. I grieve daily over the estrangement of my older daughter, Bianca. Try to remember that the secret to your AS/NT parenting and partnering problems is not fixing everything but accepting family members for who they are: That includes accepting yourself. Learn the power of neutrality. Get stress relief through psychotherapy and vacations (family, couple and by yourself). Educate yourself as much as you can about the science behind the techniques suggested. Always seek to know and speak to your partner's good intentions. As your consciousness about your unique mixed-class family grows, you may experience a paradigm shift—the sense of freedom that comes from letting go of beliefs about the way it should be and accepting the blessings of the life you have.

Let's review what we have learned. In Part One there are descriptions of typical life in mixed-class families. In Chapter One, "Helicopter Mother," you followed me from helicoptering to humility as a bewildered parent of my lovely AS daughter, Bianca. In Chapter Two, "Not-So-Ordinary Moments," I introduced you to the mind-numbing life of those not-so-ordinary moments that just shut down communication and make NTs feel oppressed by their Aspies. In Chapter Three, "What's an NT Dad Supposed to Do?," I explored the dilemma of being an NT Dad trying to rear his children with an Aspie mom, who lacks empathic maternal nurturing qualities.

Part Two covered some important theories to help expand your frame of reference for the AS/NT life, because I believe that knowledge is power. In Chapter Four, "Empathy Imbalance," I outlined Adam Smith's Empathy Imbalance Hypothesis, a simple way to understand a major communication problem. In Chapter Five, "Out of Brain - Out of Mind," I attempted to educate the reader about Simon Baron-Cohen's research into the latest developments in neuro-science, especially empathy disorders and zero degrees of empathy. In Chapter Six, "The Rules of Engagement," I brought the AS theories under the over-arching umbrella of Dialectical Psychology. I also elaborated on the intriguing concept of *context blindness*, as defined by the groundbreaking research of Peter Vermeulen. It was in this chapter that I outlined the rules of engagement, a method for resolving the problems of parenting with a spouse or partner with Asperger Syndrome.

In Part Three, I offered examples of some major problems in AS/NT families and suggested concrete ways to use the rules of engagement for resolution. In Chapter Seven, "Hapa Aspie," I emphasized the dilemmas of growing up NT with one Aspie and one NT parent. The rules of engagement require that these NT children have their own psychologist, so they can get clarity on the conflicting elements in their mixed-class family. In Chapter Eight, "Bullied or Bully," the reader was confronted with the harsh reality that, as traumatized as Aspies are, they also are the cause of emotional trauma, particularly to their own family members. We absolutely need rules of engagement for bullies whether they are NT or Aspie. In Chapter Nine, "Are You Invisible?," I familiarized the reader with the phenomenon that occurs with children and adults who live in a mixed-class family: If you are to break free of the oppression that comes from the empathy disorder of Asperger Syndrome, you must stop being invisible and take back your life. In Chapter Ten, "Can You Teach Love?," I pondered the deep question of just what love is and how to experience it with your child. Again the rules of engagement help.

In Part Four, I bring the book to a close, integrating all of the lessons learned earlier. Chapter Eleven, "The Power of Intention," underscores that all of the theories and all of the techniques mentioned in this book have no impact without good intention. Assuming that your partner has good intentions and learning to speak to those intentions is the key to successfully navigating the terrain of AS/NT parenting partnerships. Now in Chapter Twelve, "Conclusion: A New Agenda," it is time to bring the book to a finish—even though there is so much additional material to explore. In this last chapter I hope I have stirred up your curiosity to learn more. Despite the exciting discoveries touched on in this book, AS/NT relationships are still quite a mystery. One thing I am sure of: We are all connected.

Thank you for joining me on this roller coaster adventure. I hope you have learned some things that will help you understand yourself, not just your Aspies, better. I know that I understand myself better for having written it. I also fervently hope that you leave with new tools for parenting with a partner with Asperger Syndrome. I hope that the theoretical foundation you now have will help you to develop a partnering and parenting plan suited to you and your loved ones.

Throughout this book I have revealed many of my triumphs and failures. Now that the book is completed, I think I can forgive myself for my mistakes as a parent and a partner. I think I can forgive my Aspies for all of their tantrums and oppression, because those traits are balanced by their marvelous gifts to me. I think I can forgive my friends and acquaintances for their innocent generalizations about the AS/NT life. You notice that I say, "I think." I think it is because there is still more to unfold in my development as an NT child of an AS mother, as a parent to and a former parenting partner of an AS and an NT child. This is not a bad way to end this roller coaster journey—with a ticket to ride another day when there will be other surprises waiting around the corners.

One final note: I want all of you to know that you are not alone. Please feel free to contact me and share your story. I promise to write back.

You can reach me in the following ways:
- By phone at (360) 256-0448 or (503) 222-6678;
- By e-mail at info@Kmarshack.com;
- On Facebook at https://www.facebook.com/Kathy.Marshack.Ph.D;
- On Linked In as Kathy Marshack;
- On Twitter at info@kmarshack.com;
- By writing to P.O. Box 873429, Vancouver, WA 98687-3429.

Through my website, www.Kmarshack.com, you can:
- Sign up for my newsletter;
- Learn about my Meetup group for Asperger Syndrome Partners & Family of Adults with ASD;
- Download a free chapter from, or order, my first book, *Going Over the Edge*;
- View videos about Asperger relationships.

Afterword

Dr. Marshack facilitates a Meetup group devoted to those in relationships with Asperger Syndrome adults. People from all over the world participate via the web while many in the Portland, Oregon area gather in person.

The Meetup discussions, meant to enlighten, educate and embolden while offering relief and support, cover topics such as:

"How do I handle the loneliness?"
"Women with ASD."
"Empathy disorder explains it all."
"How do I tell my spouse I think they have Asperger's?"
"Is divorce the answer?"
"How do I handle the verbal abuse?"

For more information about this dynamic Meetup group, now in its fourth year, visit www.Kmarshack.com.

To give you a glimpse into the Meetup group, here are some comments from members. The names and locations are withheld for privacy.

❖ "Thank you for all the warmth and reflection. A dose of human medicine for the strung-out."

❖ "Wow! The information, love, and support to be had by attending this group are amazing. Please go if you even think you might be struggling with similar issues. You will be amazed at how much better you feel at the end of the meeting. You are NOT alone."

❖ "Great meeting! Always leave more empowered than when I came. Never a waste of time!"

❖ "There is also a most welcome social aspect for those people whose social lives have become limited as a result of accommodating their AS family members."

❖ "The one or two male voices are invaluable, as they add perspective and information. Thank you, thank you, thank you for a much-needed resource and, let's face it, a place to vent!"

❖ "I am learning to live and let go. Understanding is power. The love, acceptance and support I receive has been transforming."

❖ "This website is a lifeline to NT sanity!"

❖ "This group has given me hope, showed me ways to cope and given me my life back. I felt so alone and helpless until I found this group. It is a godsend."

"Asperger's is real, and you aren't crazy. Come to this Meetup and get some backing for your reality—and some support from others who know the game." — Dr. Kathy Marshack

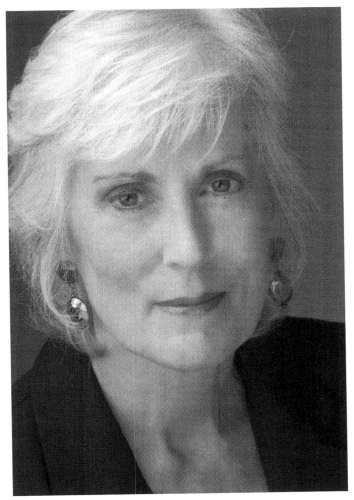

Kathy J. Marshack, Ph.D., P.S., is a licensed psychologist with more than 33 years of experience as a marriage and family therapist and business coach.

Dr. Marshack's first book on Asperger Syndrome, *Going Over the Edge? Life with a Partner or Spouse with Asperger Syndrome,* was published in 2009. After its release, she was overwhelmed by the response of readers from around the world, who felt alone and misunderstood navigating innately complex relationships with loved ones with Asperger Syndrome. In response, Dr. Marshack organized the international Meetup group, *Asperger Syndrome: Partners & Family of Adults with ASD,* which gives members the opportunity to offer support via the online forum or in-person meetings. She also blogs regularly about Asperger relationships and plans to offer webinars, so that more people can get the education and support they need.

In addition to working with those who have Asperger Syndrome, Dr. Marshack helps clients with a wide range of issues. Her expertise includes: depression, marital counseling, high-conflict divorce, codependency and adoptive family issues. She is also considered a national expert on families in business, having authored a "Families in Business" column and the book, *Entrepreneurial Couples: Making It at Work and at Home.*

Dr. Marshack and her books have been featured in articles in dozens of publications, including the *Boston Globe, Kiplinger's, The New York Times, The San Francisco Examiner, Smart Money Magazine, Inc. Magazine, USA Today* and *Business Week.* She is frequently profiled by national and local media – such as *CNN, The Lifetime Channel* and *National Public Radio.* She was also a contributor to the nationally acclaimed book, *Sixty Things to Do When You Turn Sixty.*

Dr. Marshack's credentials include a Bachelor of Science Degree in Psychology from Portland State University in Oregon, a Master's Degree in Social Work from the University of Hawaii in Hawaii, and a Doctorate in Psychology from the Fielding Institute in California. She is a Certified Practitioner of

Neurolinguistic Programming, Ericksonian Hypnosis, Thought Field Therapy and NET (Neuro-Emotional Technique). She resides by the beautiful Columbia River in Vancouver, Washington and has an office there as well as a satellite office in Portland, Oregon.

Made in the USA
Middletown, DE
21 July 2015